GOOD KIDS BAD HABITS

GOOD KIDS BAD HABITS

The RealAge® Guide to Raising Healthy Children

Jennifer Trachtenberg, M.D.

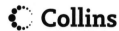

An Imprint of HarperCollinsPublishers

To my children: Noah, Eric, and Emily
I wish for you happiness, love, and healthy habits in the years ahead

This book contains advice and information relating to health care for children. It is not intended to replace medical advice and should be used to supplement rather than replace regular care by your child's pediatrician. Since every child is different, you should consult your child's pediatrician on questions specific to your child.

While certain sections of the book contain advice for dealing with emergencies when a doctor is not available, it is recommended that you seek your child's pediatrician's advice whenever possible and that you consult with him or her before embarking on any medical program or treatment.

FIRST EDITION

Designed by Nancy Singer Olaguera/ISPN Publishing Services

Library of Congress Cataloging-in-Publication Data is available upon request.

ISBN   0-06-112775-2

---

07 08 09 10 11 ISPN/RRD 10 9 8 7 6 5 4 3 2 1

CONTENTS

FOREWORD

*EDITOR'S NOTE: Mike Roizen and Mehmet Oz are America's new favorite physicians, thanks to their phenomenal bestsellers—*YOU: The Owner's Manual *and* YOU: On a Diet—*and their unforgettable TV appearances, including the show where they explained everything anyone ever wanted to know about poop (like: it should be s-shaped). Poop is a subject they've had plenty of experience with—not only as doctors, but as diaper-changing dads. Dr. Roizen has two kids, Jeff and Jenny, and Dr. Oz has four, Daphne, Arabella, Zoe, and Oliver.*

As doctors, we both see the long-term effects of good kids with bad habits virtually every time we go into the operating room. The patients we treat get younger and younger, but their bodies' biological ages—or RealAges—are older and older. Clogged arteries, high blood pressure, diabetic complications, flabby muscles, and joints stressed by obesity are practically a given.

As dads, we have worked to protect our own kids from today's overeating, underexercising lifestyle. But we discovered firsthand what every parent knows: It isn't easy. Which is why *Good Kids, Bad Habits* was written. Like us, Dr. Trachtenberg—who has three children of her own—knows that parents need every morsel of help they can get to convince kids to put down the remote, pass up the cookies, grab an apple, and go for a bike ride. Both of us learned similar lessons along the hectic six-lane highway we took to raise our children.

Still, knowing what kids should do has always been less tricky than getting them to actually do it. How many parents do you know who have great intentions, yet somehow their kids veer way off course? That's why when Mike's first child, Jeffrey, was nine months old, his wife persuaded him—OK, forced him—to take a course called Parent Effectiveness Training. But he says today that it turned out to be one of the best courses he ever took, because it taught him how to communicate with kids and, yes, certain patients, who really don't want to hear what their dad, or doctor, is saying.

From that class, from our own parents, and simply from being dads—though there's nothing simple about fatherhood!—we wound up figuring out five principles that really help kids form good habits for life.

1. Make "can't" a four-letter word.
2. Figure out who owns the problem and has to solve it.
3. Be a positive role model.
4. Do fun, healthy things together.
5. Stick up for your siblings and your friends.

First, try to guide the kids toward activities that they *can* do, where they'll shine, and then always hand out compliments whenever they do something well or simply kind. Like Mike saying to his daughter, "Jenny, it was terrific of you to stop and help that man across the street, especially when you were worried about being late for dance class."

Second, and a critical important foundation for good habits, is to tell children (and others) the truth about who owns a problem. This example is a bit dramatic, but it's a real one Mike had with his son: "Jeff, if you don't wear your bike helmet and you get hit by a car, you could end up so brain-damaged that you couldn't play baseball or even turn on the TV. You might not have enough gray matter left to care, but it would destroy me to see you in the hospital for the rest of your life. So do *me* a favor: Wear your helmet." In the end, Mike (like other parents) owned the helmet problem because ultimately he'd have to cope with the results of his son not wearing one.

But here's a problem Jeff owned. His dad said to him, "Good bet that eating those cheese-smothered fries will keep you off the team because they'll slow you down—their artery-clogging effects will keep your muscles from getting enough blood." That one was Jeff's decision to make. Guess what he did! Knowing when they own a problem lets kids be responsible for their own choices. And yes, sometimes they'll make as many bad bets as a drunken gambler, but overall they'll gradually take responsibility for healthy choices.

It's important to package all this advice with love, of course. Kids may blow off your brilliant insights, even at the risk of a battle, but if the insights are offered with love, the battle will blow over pretty easily. And the advice may save them later on.

Adults also have to lead by example. Try to be a role model for good health habits, from exercise to eating—like choosing walnuts over chips or tomato sauce over mayonnaise. For instance, instead of watching sports on TV, play games with your kids and try to make it so much fun that it keeps them coming back for more. Mehmet and his brood are currently crazy for ball tag, which pits him against them. He runs around kicking a soccer ball, and anyone the ball touches has to freeze. The other kids can release the freeze by tagging him with their hands, but if Mehmet freezes all of the kids before they tag each other, he wins. Naturally, the game is all about beating dad, so there's nonstop running, yelling, and laughing. But because it's a huge workout, it's a win every time.

Remember that much of what kids learn about food, fitness, tattoos, sports, sex, sleep, homework, piercing—you name it—doesn't come from you. It comes from other kids. Having a health-conscious older sibling, or cool kid next door whom the kids look up to, can be a godsend. Oz's eldest, Daphne, is both cool and takes great care of herself. Not only do her sibs admire her but she's so smart about health that she wrote a whole book about it at age nineteen. And his eleven-year-old, Zoe, is the family athlete. She drags seven-year-old Oliver to every game she goes to, and now he's as hooked on sports as she is.

Finally, teach kids to stick up for each other and their friends. When they give someone else a boost, the other kid feels good, they feel good—and the favor usually gets returned.

Those five guidelines should help your kids, like ours, form good habits and avoid bad ones. They give kids a sense of self-esteem and responsibility, a live-in role model, the knowledge that health can be fun, and a foundation for lifelong trusting relationships.

But the best thing we ever did for our kids was to choose great moms. Jenny and Jeff Roizen are now young adults and doing great, but Mike's the first one to say that's due much more to Nancy's influence than his—that her constant guidance instilled good habits in their children, and that she's the one who really taught them about setting goals. Lisa Oz, like Nancy, is a natural at knowing how to encourage kids to achieve anything they want to, and has been figuring out ways to instill healthy habits since they were toddlers. Both of us got to see their moms' greatness firsthand, and the habits they instilled stand our kids in good stead every day.

INTRODUCTION

Here's why *Good Kids, Bad Habits* was written: to protect our children's health future. Kids today have developed so many bad health habits that they're facing heart attacks *in their 30s*. Experts predict they'll be the first generation of children to have a lower life expectancy than their parents.

The number one defense against this is you, their parents. Pediatricians can help, but nobody has more influence over kids than parents. You can stop it. How?

This book will give you the tools you need, beginning with the unique RealAge Healthy Kids Test. It will tell you just where your kids are headed healthwise—the good news and the bad. Then it will show you, step by step, exactly how to give your kids the best possible shot at great health and happiness in the years ahead. Nothing—nothing—is more important.

I can already see the worry furrow on your forehead. Don't panic. When I talk about bad habits, I'm not talking about skipping a bath or eating a bowl of Chunky Monkey for dinner on a special occasion. I'm talking about the day-to-day stuff. The stuff good health is made of: enjoying a wide variety of tasty foods, making time for active fun and games, and avoiding accidents.

With the RealAge Healthy Kids plan, you can:

- Lower your child's risk of diabetes, heart disease, osteo-porosis, and asthma.
- Increase your child's focus, energy, and creativity.
- Boost your child's emotional health and social skills.
- Reduce your child's risk of serious injuries and accidents.

In addition, you'll learn how to deal with ongoing challenges such as allergies and food intolerances, and manage psychological issues, including ADHD, anxiety, and depression. You'll also see more smiles, fewer tears, and many happier, healthier days.

It all comes down to establishing good habits and breaking bad ones. The earlier, the better, of course—but it's as true for kids as it is for adults that it's *never* too late to start.

As a pediatrician, I've worked long and hard with the parents and children who visit my office, but that's the proverbial drop in the bucket. I desperately wanted to find a way to share with a larger audience everything I've learned about developing the habits that improve a child's chances at a happy, healthy future.

That's why I teamed up with RealAge—creator of the Real-Age® test (more about this in a moment) and an innovator in improving health habits in adults—and shared my efforts to reach out to parents via the Internet, TV, radio, and magazine articles.

The RealAge experts knew they could help kids change bad habits to good ones because they've already done it for adults. More than 15 million people have taken the original RealAge test and been inspired to improve their diet, exercise, and wellness habits. The test calculates your biological age, based on everything from genetics to how well you've taken care of your body. So if the calendar says you're 42 but you take good care of yourself, your body might only be 35. Conversely, if you don't take care of yourself, you could be aging faster than average and have a 50-year-old body.* Motivating, isn't it!

But that's not all. Along the way, the RealAge team discovered that a large percentage of unhealthy adults had developed poor lifestyle habits in childhood.

Personally, I couldn't bear to read any more shocking statistics like these:

- The number of kids who are medically obese has doubled—and in some groups tripled—since 1980.
- About 25 percent of obese children grow into obese adults.
- An astonishing 75 percent of overweight children become overweight adults.

The suggestions I'll give you to prevent this from happening are the same ones I give my patients. They're based on a combination of my years of pediatric experience and the latest medical research. Some are tried and true; some may surprise you, though I won't ask you to do anything strange or difficult. You don't have to take your kids trekking in the mountains, or get them to eat liver or give up ice cream. Instead, we'll take small steps together—but ones that can have a huge, lifelong impact on a child's health and happiness. I'll even show you how to get kids to choose healthy foods at the grocery store . . . at a very young age!

Just the fact that you're reading this book tells me two things: First, that you're aware of the quicksand so many kids are sinking into today, particularly problems triggered by obesity and inactivity. Second, that you're a proactive parent. Parents like

---

* Fortunately, while birthdays aren't reversible, your biological age is. For how to grow younger and healthier, go to www.realage.com.

you give pediatricians like me great hope. Because while you rely on your pediatrician to keep your children healthy, we rely on you as well. The quality of a child's health care depends on the partnership among pediatrician, parent, and—after a certain age—the child. The three of us are in it together.

How healthy are your child's habits? Let's find out.

The Really Scary Stuff:
Kids Are Getting Adult Diseases

If you don't get involved, your kids could soon be facing this frightening list of what used to be adults-only health problems.

Kids with High Blood Pressure Here's who's at risk: Kids who spend hours on the couch watching TV or playing video games. Kids who eat poorly. Kids who weigh too much. Kids who are under a lot of stress. And here's what chronic high blood pressure can do to kids (and adults): damage their kidneys, eyes, brains, and hearts.

Kids with Clogged Arteries Early signs of atherosclerosis—including the buildup of fatty plaques in arteries—are now being seen in kids as young as 12. One study found that the arteries of obese kids resemble those of middle-aged smokers. Even mildly overweight children are vulnerable, and the risk rises as the pounds do.

Kids Who Can't Breathe Recent studies have made a strong connection between obesity and asthma (as well as between asthma and pollutants, such as secondhand smoke). Worse, because asthma limits activity, and inactivity ups obesity, a vicious cycle quickly forms.

Kids with Syndrome X Also known as metabolic syndrome, this is a cluster of conditions—from high blood pressure to high triglycerides and insulin resistance—that frequently leads to diabetes and heart disease, among other problems. Studies suggest that 12 percent of all children in the United States and up to 30 percent of obese children now have syndrome X.

Kids with Weak Bones Building strong bones early in life is critical, but it takes regular exercise and a balanced, mineral-rich diet. Without both, children's skeletons do not develop properly, and their bones are more likely to fracture now and later.

Kids with Self-Esteem Problems It's not news that children can be cruel. But fat kids are especially prone to getting teased, bullied, and rejected. Years of being socially isolated can turn low self-esteem into full-blown depression.

Kids Who Can't Sleep, Can't Focus, and Can't Learn Kids who don't eat well and don't exercise have erratic sleep patterns, so they end up cranky and tired. They learn to compensate by chugging caffeine-spiked (and calorie-loaded) sodas and energy drinks all day to keep them awake, but then they can't fall asleep at night. And so it goes.

Kids Who Get Sick a Lot It's the same story: Inactive, overweight children with unbalanced diets have more respiratory illnesses—colds, flu, asthma—than slimmer, more active kids.

Chapter 1

TAKE THE TEST
How Healthy Are Your Child's Habits? Take the RealAge Healthy Kids Test and Find Out

I imagine you've got this book balanced on your knee at an "in between" moment—in between dropping off and picking up your kids, in between dinner and bedtime, in between laundry and playtime. And you're thinking, *Yeah, right, Dr. Jen, of course, I want to be a better parent, a better role model, but where the heck do I begin?*

Got a pencil? First, let's figure out how healthy your child's habits are with the RealAge Healthy Kids Test. If you have more than one child, use different colored pencils or pens; kids' habits aren't the same, even when they live in the same house.

Okay, here's how the test works. A series of questions probes how well you and your child are working together as a team to establish good habits in areas ranging from overall health and nutrition to fitness and safety. For each section you'll get a score between 1 and 10; average those scores to get your overall score. The higher it is, the better you're doing as a parent, and the better your child's potential is to be healthy now—and for years to come. (To have all the calculations done for you, go to www.RealAge.com/parenting and take the test online.)

Just remember that this one-of-a-kind test looks at health *habits,* not actual health. It assesses only things you and your child can control. A preexisting health problem—say, asthma— won't hurt your score; however, not properly managing this condition could lower it.

Once you know each child's score, you can predict—and this part might make you both excited and a little nervous— what your child's RealAge will be as an adult. As I said earlier, RealAge is the biological age of a person's body, which is heavily based on how well it's maintained. The healthy habits that are established now in many ways can predict your child's health and life expectancy. That's why this test is so important.

Also, try to update your child's test score every ninety days (and redo your own RealAge test regularly, too). That way, you can monitor the progress your child *and* you are making and identify any problem areas that need attention.

So, let's get going on the reason we're both here—giving your child the best chance possible for a long, healthy, and happy life.

The RealAge Healthy Kids Test

Section 1: General Health and Medical Conditions

	Rattle	Bear	Backpack
1. How well do you feel you and your child are doing in terms of establishing lifelong healthy habits? a. Excellent b. Very well c. Average d. Not so well e. Poor	a. 10 b. 7 c. 5 d. 3 e. 0	a. 10 b. 7 c. 5 d. 3 e. 0	a. 10 b. 7 c. 5 d. 3 e. 0
2. Is your child up to date on all recommended vaccinations? a. Yes b. No c. Not sure d. Not all, due to health conditions/concerns	**RATTLE** a. 10 b. 0 c. 5 d. 5	**BEAR** a. 10 b. 0 c. 5 d. 5	**BACKPACK** a. 10 b. 0 c. 5 d. 5

NOTE: Throughout, "NA" means "not applicable"

3. Please check any of the following health issues that apply to your child:	No points (see follow-up question)

3. Please check any of the following health issues that apply to your child:

   a.　ADHD

   b.　Allergies or sinus problems

   c.　Asthma

   d.　Autism

   e.　Behavioral problems

   f.　Blindness

   g.　Cancer

   h.　Cystic fibrosis

   i.　Depression or anxiety

   j.　Diabetes

   k.　Down syndrome

   l.　Eczema

   m.　Frequent urinary tract infections

   n.　GERD

   o.　Hearing impairment

   p.　High blood pressure

   q.　Iron deficiency

   r.　Juvenile rheumatoid arthritis

   s.　Physical disability

   t.　Sickle cell anemia

   u.　Sleep disorder

   v.　Other

   w.　None of the above (skip next question)

4. Are you and your child managing the conditions you checked by visiting a doctor or other specialist? a. Yes, for all checked conditions b. Yes, for some conditions c. No	RATTLE a. 10 b. 10 c. 0	BEAR a. 10 b. 10 c. 0	BACKPACK a. 10 b. 10 c. 0
5. Has your child had one or more routine checkup(s) this year? a Yes b. No c. Not sure	RATTLE a. 10 b. 2 c. 2 d. 2	BEAR a. 7 b. 4 c. 2 d. 2	BACKPACK a. 10 b. 10 c. 5 d. 5

Add up all your points and write the total in the box.

Section 1 Total Points:

Section 2: Nutrition

1. How many times per week does your child eat breakfast? a. Every day b. 4 to 6 days c. 2 to 3 days d. Never (skip next question)	RATTLE a. 8 b. 0 c. 0 d. 0	BEAR a. 8 b. 4 c. 1 d. 0	BACKPACK a. 8 b. 5 c. 2 d. 0

2. What does your child typically eat for breakfast? (choose up to 2)	RATTLE	BEAR	BACKPACK
a. Sweetened cereal	a. 3	a. 3	a. 5
b. Prepackaged breakfast bar or donuts	b. 1	b. 3	b. 4
c. Eggs	c. 5	c. 5	c. 5
d. Yogurt	d. 8	d. 8	d. 8
e. Whole-grain cereal or whole-grain toast	e. 8	e. 8	e. 8
f. Whole-grain Os	f. 7	f. 7	f. 7
g. Jarred baby food or baby cereal	g. 9	g. NA	g. NA
h. Hot cereal or oatmeal	h. 8	h. 8	h. 8
i. Milk	i. 10	i. 10	i. 10
j. Breast milk	j. 10	j. NA	j. NA
k. Juice	k. 8	k. 8	k. 8
l. Fruit	l. 8	l. 8	l. 8
m. Pancakes	m. 5	m. 5	m. 5
n. Other foods not mentioned	n. 5	n. 5	n. 5
o. Not sure	o. 0	o. 0	o. 0

3. Overall, how balanced and varied do you consider your child's diet?	RATTLE	BEAR	BACKPACK
a. Very balanced and varied	a. 10	a. 10	a. 10
b. Somewhat	b. 6	b. 7	b. 7
c. Not very	c. 1	c. 1	c. 4
d. Not sure	d. 1	d. 1	d. 5

4. Which kinds of protein foods does your child eat fairly regularly? (choose up to 3)	RATTLE	BEAR	BACKPACK
a. Hamburgers or beef	a. 0	a. 4	a. 5
b. Hot dogs	b. 0	b. 0 (if under age 4)	b. 4
c. Fish	c. 7		c. 8
d. Lunch meat	d. 4	c. 8	d. 4
e. Sausage and bacon	e. 4	d. 4	e. 4
f. Poultry	f. 6	e. 4	f. 6
g. Pork	g. 6	f. 6	g. 6
h. Meat alternatives, such as soy burgers	h. 5	g. 6	h. 5
i. Deep-fried protein foods (chicken nuggets, fish sticks, etc.)	i. 0	h. 5	i. 0
j. None of the above	j. 5	i. 0	j. 5
		j. 5	

5. What are typical snacks for your child?	RATTLE	BEAR	BACKPACK
(choose up to 3)	a. 10	a. 10	a. 10
a. Fresh fruit	b. 5	b. 5	b. 5
b. Fruit roll-ups	c. 5	c. 5	c. 5
c. Cookies	d. 3	d. 3	d. 3
d. Candy	e. 5	e. 5	e. 5
e. Crackers or pretzels	f. 3	f. 3	f. 3
f. Chips (regular)	g. 5	g. 5	g. 5
g. Chips (baked)	h. 7	h. 7	h. 7
h. Yogurt	i. 7	i. 7	i. 7
i. Cheese	j. 5	j. 5	j. 5
j. Bread	k. 8	k. 2	k. 7
k. Raw vegetables, such as carrots, celery, or broccoli	l. 6	l. 6	l. 6
l. Nuts	m. 5	m. 5	m. 5
m. Other	n. 5	n. 5	n. 5
n. None of the above			

6. What does your child drink often? (choose up to 3)	RATTLE	BEAR	BACKPACK
a. 100% fruit/vegetable juice	a. 5	a. 10	a. 10
b. Juice drinks (not 100% juice)	b. 6	b. 6	b. 6
c. Powdered punch or lemonade	c. 5	c. 5	c. 5
d. Flavored soft drinks or soda	d. 1	d. 1	d. 1
e. Sports drinks such as Gatorade	e. 5	e. 5	e. 5
f. Water	f. 10	f. 10	f. 10
g. Milk or soy-based milk products	g. 10	g. 10	g. 10
h. Breast milk	h. 10	h. NA	h. NA
i. Chocolate milk	i. 5	i. 5	i. 5
j. None of the above	j. 5	j. 5	j. 5

7. Does your child eat 5 to 9 servings daily of vegetables and fruits?	RATTLE	BEAR	BACKPACK
a. Yes, always	a. 10	a. 10	a. 10
b. Yes, most of the time	b. 5	b. 6	b. 8
c. No	c. 0	c. 0	c. 0
d. Not sure	d. 0	d. 0	d. 0

8. Does your child eat well-balanced bagged lunches—with a variety of foods from all food groups—or school-provided lunches?	RATTLE	BEAR	BACKPACK
a. Bagged lunches always	a. NA	a. 8	a. 8
b. Bagged lunches most of the time	b. NA	b. 7	b. 7
c. School lunches always	c. NA	c. 3	c. 3
d. School lunches most of the time	d. NA	d. 4	d. 4
e. Half bagged, half school lunches	e. NA	e. 5	e. 5
f. Skips lunches	f. NA	f. 1	f. 1
g. Not in school yet	g. NA	g. 5	g. NA
h. Don't know	h. NA	h. 4	h. 5

9. How often does your child eat sweets?	RATTLE	BEAR	BACKPACK
a. At every meal	a. 0	a. 0	a. 0
b. Occasionally as a snack or for dessert	b. 5	b. 5	b. 5
c. Only on special occasions	c. 5	c. 5	c. 5
d. Never	d. 6	d. 6	d. 6
e. Don't know	e. 3	e. 3	e. 5

10. Does your child regularly take a multivitamin?	RATTLE	BEAR	BACKPACK
a. Yes	a. NA	a. 6	a. 6
b. No	b. NA	b. 5	b. 5
c. Not sure	c. NA	c. 0	c. 0

11. How many times per month does your child help pick out healthy foods for dinner, such as fruits and vegetables? a. Always b. Most of the time c. Sometimes d. Hardly ever e. Never	RATTLE	BEAR	BACKPACK
	a. NA	a. 8	a. 8
	b. NA	b. 7	b. 7
	c. NA	c. 6	c. 6
	d. NA	d. 5	d. 5
	e. NA	e. 4	e. 4
12. Does your child help in meal preparation? (choose up to 2) a. Helps wash vegetables and fruit b. Sets the timer, microwave c. Helps in dessert preparation d. Decides what we will have e. Stirs the food f. Sets the table g. Does not help	RATTLE	BEAR	BACKPACK
	a. NA	a. 6	a. 6
	b. NA	b. 6	b. 6
	c. NA	c. 6	c. 6
	d. NA	d. 6	d. 6
	e. NA	e. 6	e. 6
	f. NA	f. 6	f. 6
	g. NA	g. 4	g. 4
13. How often do you sit down and eat together as a family? a. Never, we don't have time b. 1 to 3 days per week c. 4 to 6 days per week d. 7 days per week	RATTLE	BEAR	BACKPACK
	a. 0	a. 3	a. 3
	b. 1	b. 6	b. 6
	c. 5	c. 7	c. 7
	d. 8	d. 8	d. 8

14. Where does your child most often eat dinner? (choose 1)	RATTLE	BEAR	BACKPACK
a. At the dinner table or kitchen bar, with family or friends	a. 6	a. 9	a. 9
	b. 4	b. 4	b. 5
b. At the dinner table or kitchen bar, alone	c. 2	c. 2	c. 5
c. On the go (in the car or other nondining area)	d. 3	d. 4	d. 4
d. At a restaurant	e. 1	e. 3	e. 3
e. In front of the TV	f. 1	f. 3	f. 5
f. In his/her room	g. 0	g. 0	g. 4
g. Don't know			

Add up all your points and write the total in the box.

Section 2 Total Points: [ ]

Section 3: Physical and Mental Exercise

1. What is the total time per day your child spends watching TV or movies, or playing video games?	RATTLE	BEAR	BACKPACK
a. 0 to 1 hour	a. 4	a. 5	a. 5
b. 1 to 3 hours	b. 1	b. 2	b. 2
c. More than 3 hours	c. 0	c. 0	c. 0

2. How much time does your child spend each day using the computer for things other than school projects? a. Never b. Less than an hour c. 1 hour d. 2 hours e. 3 hours or more f. Don't know	RATTLE	BEAR	BACKPACK
	a. NA	a. 7	a. 7
	b. NA	b. 6	b. 6
	c. NA	c. 5	c. 5
	d. NA	d. 4	d. 4
	e. NA	e. 3	e. 3
	f. NA	f. 1	f. 1
3. Is your child supervised (by an adult or by software) when using the Internet? a. Yes, always b. Yes, most of the time c. No d. Does not use the Internet	RATTLE	BEAR	BACKPACK
	a. NA	a. 8	a. 8
	b. NA	b. 5	b. 5
	c. NA	c. 3	c. 3
	d. NA	d. 5	d. 5
4. Does your child have a special area in the home to do homework? a. Yes, at the kitchen or dining table b. Yes, at a desk in the bedroom c. Yes, on the family room floor or at the coffee table d. No, does homework anywhere and everywhere e. No, does homework in the car or bus f. No, doesn't have homework g. No, is not in school yet	RATTLE	BEAR	BACKPACK
	a. NA	a. 10	a. 10
	b. NA	b. 8	b. 8
	c. NA	c. 8	c. 8
	d. NA	d. 4	d. 4
	e. NA	e. 5	e. 5
	f. NA	f. 5	f. 0
	g. NA	g. 5	g. NA

5. When does your child do homework?	RATTLE	BEAR	BACKPACK
a. Right after school	a. NA	a. 4	a. 4
b. After sports/activities	b. NA	b. 7	b. 7
c. After dinner	c. NA	c. 6	c. 6
d. In the morning, before school	d. NA	d. 5	d. 5
e. Don't know	e. NA	e. 1	e. 1
f. Doesn't have homework	f. NA	f. NA	f. 1

6. How does your child spend leisure time? (choose up to 2)	RATTLE	BEAR	BACKPACK
a. Watching TV	a. 0	a. 1	a. 3
b. Playing video games	b. 0	b. 1	b. 4
c. Using the computer	c. 0	c. 4	c. 5
d. Reading	d. 8	d. 10	d. 10
e. Doing arts and crafts	e. NA	e. 8	e. 8
f. Playing in his/her room	f. 7	f. 7	f. 7
g. Playing actively outdoors	g. 8	g. 10	g. 10
h. Playing actively indoors (gym, rink, etc.)	h. 7	h. 9	h. 9
i. Other	i. 5	i. 5	i. 5

7. Which clubs, activities, or organizations does your child participate in regularly? (choose up to 2) a. School sports/clubs b. Baseball, soccer, or other organized sport group c. Music or dance lessons or theater/drama club d. Scouting group e. Religious studies or community groups f. Other g. None of the above	**RATTLE** a. NA b. NA c. NA d. NA e. NA f. NA g. NA	**BEAR** a. 9 b. 9 c. 9 d. 9 e. 8 f. 5 g. 1	**BACKPACK** a. 9 b. 9 c. 9 d. 9 e. 8 f. 5 g. 1
8. What is your child's most frequent mode of transportation? (choose 1) a. Walking b. Stroller c. Being carried d. Bike e. Skateboard f. Scooter g. In-line or roller skates h. Car, bus, or subway i. Other j. None of the above	**RATTLE** a. 10 b. 5 c. 5 d. NA e. NA f. NA g. NA h. NA i. NA j. 5	**BEAR** a. 10 b. NA c. NA d. 9 e. 8 f. 7 g. 8 h. 5 i. 5 j. 5	**BACKPACK** a. 10 b. NA c. NA d. 9 e. 8 f. 7 g. 8 h. 5 i. 5 j. 5

9. Which activities does your child enjoy most frequently? (choose up to 2)	RATTLE	BEAR	BACKPACK
a. Walking	a. 7	a. 7	a. 7
b. Camping	b. 7	b. 7	b. 7
c. Playing video games	c. 3	c. 3	c. 3
d. Going to amusement parks	d. 4	d. 4	d. 4
e. Hiking	e. 8	e. 8	e. 8
f. Visiting museums, aquariums, or zoos	f. 6	f. 6	f. 6
g. Swimming	g. 9	g. 9	g. 9
h. Shopping	h. 5	h. 5	h. 5
i. Completing household chores or projects	i. 6	i. 6	i. 6
j. Gardening	j. 8	j. 8	j. 8
k. Working on hobby projects or games	k. 5	k. 5	k. 5
l. Watching movies	l. 2	l. 2	l. 2
m. None of the above	m. 2	m. 2	m. 2
n. Other	n. 5	n. 5	n. 5

Add up all your points and write the total in the box.

Section 3 Total Points:

Section 4: Personal Care

1. How often does your child brush his/her teeth?	RATTLE	BEAR	BACKPACK
a. 3 times per day	a. 7	a. 7	a. 7
b. 2 times per day	b. 4	b. 4	b. 4
c. Once a day	c. 2	c. 2	c. 2
d. A few times per week	d. 0	d. 0	d. 0
e. Never	e. 0	e. 0	e. 0
f. Don't know	f. 0	f. 4	f. 5
2. How often does your child floss?	RATTLE	BEAR	BACKPACK
a. 3 times per day	a. NA	a. 8	a. 8
b. 2 times per day	b. NA	b. 8	b. 8
c. Once a day	c. NA	c. 8	c. 8
d. A few times per week	d. NA	d. 4	d. 4
e. Never	e. NA	e. 1	e. 1
f. Don't know	f. NA	f. 4	f. 5
3. Does your child see the dentist at least once a year?	RATTLE	BEAR	BACKPACK
a. Yes	a. NA	a. 10	a. 10
b. No	b. NA	b. 3	b. 3

4. How much sleep does your child get on most nights?	RATTLE	BEAR	BACKPACK
a. 10+ hours	a. 7	a. 7	a. 6
b. 8 to 9 hours	b. 4	b. 5	b. 7
c. 6 to 7 hours	c. 0	c. 3	c. 4
d. 5 or fewer hours	d. 0	d. 0	d. 3
e. Don't know	e. 0	e. 0	e. 0

Add up all your points and write the total in the box.

Section 4 Total Points:

Section 5: Social and Emotional Health

1. Select the extended family members with whom your child maintains contact through visits, e-mail, phone calls, etc. (choose all that apply) a. Grandparents b. Aunts and uncles c. Cousins d. Close friends of the family e. Other f. None	RATTLE	BEAR	BACKPACK
a.	a. 8	a. 8	a. 8
b.	b. 8	b. 8	b. 8
c.	c. 8	c. 8	c. 8
d.	d. 8	d. 8	d. 8
e.	e. 8	e. 8	e. 8
f.	f. 2	f. 2	f. 2

2. How well does your child play with siblings and children in his/her age group? a. Very well, always b. Very well, most of the time c. Not very well d. Don't know	RATTLE	BEAR	BACKPACK
	a. NA	a. 7	a. 7
	b. NA	b. 6	b. 6
	c. NA	c. 4	c. 4
	d. NA	d. 3	d. 4

3. How well do you think your child deals with peer pressure? a. Very well—makes up his/her own mind b. Is somewhat guided by peers c. Is very influenced by peers d. Don't know	RATTLE	BEAR	BACKPACK
	a. NA	a. 7	a. 9
	b. NA	b. 6	b. 5
	c. NA	c. 4	c. 0
	d. NA	d. 5	d. 3

4. How do you think your child would rate his/her overall self-worth or self-image? a. Very high b. High c. Average d. Low e. Very low f. Don't know	RATTLE	BEAR	BACKPACK
	a. NA	a. 8	a. 9
	b. NA	b. 7	b. 8
	c. NA	c. 6	c. 7
	d. NA	d. 4	d. 4
	e. NA	e. 3	e. 0
	f. NA	f. 1	f. 0

5. Overall, how would you rate your child's confidence? a. Very high b. Average c. Low d. Very low e. Don't know	RATTLE	BEAR	BACKPACK
	a. NA	a. 8	a. 9
	b. NA	b. 6	b. 6
	c. NA	c. 4	c. 4
	d. NA	d. 3	d. 0
	e. NA	e. 1	e. 0

6. How often does your child try new activities?	RATTLE	BEAR	BACKPACK
a. Often	a. 8	a. 10	a. 10
b. Every once in a while	b. 5	b. 6	b. 6
c. Never	c. 3	c. 4	c. 5

7. How often does your child come to you for help with a problem?	RATTLE	BEAR	BACKPACK
a. Often	a. NA	a. 8	a. 8
b. Every once in a while	b. NA	b. 5	b. 5
c. Never	c. NA	c. 3	c. 4

Add up all your points and write the total in the box.

Section 5 Total Points:

Section 6: Safety Habits

1. Does your child wear appropriate protective gear (helmet, elbow and knee pads, etc.) when participating in activities such as biking , snowboarding, and contact sports?	RATTLE	BEAR	BACKPACK
a. Yes, always	a. NA	a. 10	a. 8
b. Most of the time	b. NA	b. 4	b. 5
c. No, never	c. NA	c. 0	c. 4

2. In a motor vehicle, does your child sit with the seat belt fastened correctly or, if under 4'9" tall, in a correctly attached car/booster seat? a. Yes, always b. Most of the time c. No, never d. We don't drive in vehicles	**RATTLE** a. 10 b. 3 c. 0 d. 5	**BEAR** a. 10 b. 3 c. 0 d. 5	**BACKPACK** a. 10 b. 3 c. 0 d. 5
3. Does your child sit in the backseat of the vehicle? a. Yes, always b. Most of the time c. Hardly ever d. No	**RATTLE** a. 10 b. 0 c. 0 d. 0	**RATTLE** a. 10 b. 0 c. 0 d. 0	**BACKPACK** a. NA b. NA c. NA d. NA
4. If your child drives, how confident are you about his/her skills and level of response behind the wheel? a. Very confident b. Somewhat confident c. Not very confident	**RATTLE** a. NA b. NA c. NA	**BEAR** a. NA b. NA c. NA	**BACKPACK** a. 5 b. 4 c. 0

5. Is your child monitored while taking a bath?
a. Yes, always
b. Yes, most of the time
c. No
	RATTLE
	
	a. 10
	b. 0
	c. 0
		BEAR
		
		a. If under age 6, 10;
		   if older, NA
		b. If under age 6, 0;
		   if older, NA
		c. If under age 6, 0;
		   if older, NA
			BACKPACK
			
			a. NA
			b. 0
			c. NA

6. Does your child know how to swim? a. Yes b. No, but will be taking lessons soon c. No	RATTLE a. 10 b. 5 c. 5	BEAR a. 10 b. 5 c. 0	BACKPACK a. 10 b. 5 c. 0
7. Does your child know the universal choking sign? a. Yes b. No	RATTLE a. 10 b. 5	BEAR a. 10 b. 0	BACKPACK a. 10 b. 0
8. Do you know what to do if your child is choking? a. Yes b. No	RATTLE a. 10 b. 0	BEAR a. 10 b. 0	BACKPACK a. 10 b. 0
9. Is there a first-aid kit in your home? a. Yes b. No	RATTLE a. 8 b. 3	BEAR a. 8 b. 3	BACKPACK a. 8 b. 3

10. Is your child's babysitter or day-care worker certified in CPR? a. Yes b. No c. Don't know	RATTLE a. 10 b. 0 c. 0	BEAR a. 10 b. 0 c. 0	BACKPACK a. NA b. NA c. NA
11. Does your child wear sunblock and/or sun-protective clothing when outside for an extended period of time? a. Yes, always b. Yes, most of the time c. Yes, sometimes d. Hardly ever e. No, never f. Not sure	RATTLE a. 10 b. 3 c. 2 d. 1 e. 0 f. 0	BEAR a. 10 b. 3 c. 2 d. 1 e. 0 f. 0	BACKPACK a. 10 b. 3 c. 2 d. 1 e. 0 f. 5
12. Does anyone smoke in your home? a. Yes b. Only when we have company c. No	RATTLE a. 0 b. 3 c. 10	BEAR a. 0 b. 3 c. 10	BACKPACK a. 0 b. 3 c. 10
13. Circle all that apply to your home: a. Tested for lead b. Tested for radon c. Equipped with smoke detectors d. Equipped with carbon monoxide detectors e. None of the above	RATTLE a. 10 b. 10 c. 10 d. 10 e. 0	BEAR a. 10 b. 10 c. 10 d. 10 e. 0	BACKPACK a. 10 b. 10 c. 10 d. 10 e. 0

14. Circle all that apply to your home:	RATTLE	BEAR	BACKPACK
a. Baby gates, window guards, and other protective barriers	a. 10	a. 10	a. NA
b. Locks or safety latches on cabinets that contain risky items such as cleaning agents and medicine	b. 10	b. 10	b. NA
c. Padding around hard surfaces and sharp corners	c. 10	c. 10	c. NA
d. Stoppers or plugs in electrical outlets	d. 10	d. 10	d. NA
e. Lower setting on the hot water thermostat	e. 10	e. 10	e. NA
f. None of the above	f. 0	f. 0	f. NA

Add up all your points and write the total in the box.

Section 5 Total Points:

How the Scoring Works

In the white parts of the charts below, circle your total points for each section. Next, write the corresponding score above it in the space provided. Then follow directions at the end of the charts. For example, if your total points for Section 1 were 9–11, your score would be 4.

Section 1: General Health and Medical Conditions   My Score:____

SCORE	1	2	3	4	5	6	7	8	9	10
RATTLE	0–2	3–5	6–8	9–11	12–14	15–17	18–20	21–23	24–26	27+
BEAR	0–2	3–5	6–8	9–11	12–14	15–17	18–20	21–23	24–26	27+
BACKPACK	0–2	3–5	6–8	9–11	12–14	15–17	18–20	21–23	24–26	27+

Section 2: Nutrition   My Score:_____

SCORE	1	2	3	4	5	6	7	8	9	10
RATTLE	0–20	21–33	34–46	47–58	59–71	72–84	85–96	97–108	109–120	121+
BEAR	0–15	16–31	32–48	49–63	64–78	79–93	94–108	109–123	124–138	139+
BACKPACK	0–15	16–31	32–48	49–63	64–78	79–93	94–108	109–123	124–138	139+

Section 3: Physical and Mental Exercise   My Score:_____

SCORE	1	2	3	4	5	6	7	8	9	10
RATTLE	0–5	6–10	11–16	17–21	22–27	28–33	34–39	40–45	46–57	58+
BEAR	0–11	12–22	23–33	34–44	45–55	56–66	67–77	78–88	89–99	100+
BACKPACK	0–11	12–22	23–33	34–44	45–55	56–66	67–77	78–88	89–99	100+

Section 4: Personal Care   My Score:_____

SCORE	1	2	3	4	5	6	7	8	9	10
RATTLE	NA	NA	0–1	2–3	4–5	6–7	8–9	10–11	12–13	14+
BEAR	0–2	3–6	7–10	11–14	15–18	19–22	23–25	26–28	29–31	32+
BACKPACK	0–2	3–6	7–10	11–14	15–18	19–22	23–25	26–28	29–31	32+

Section 5: Social and Emotional Health   My Score:_____

SCORE	1	2	3	4	5	6	7	8	9	10
RATTLE	0–5	6–10	11–16	17–21	22–27	28–33	34–39	40–45	46–57	58+
BEAR	0–8	9–18	19–27	28–36	37–45	46–55	56–65	66–74	75–87	88+
BACKPACK	0–8	9–18	19–27	28–36	37–45	46–55	56–65	66–74	75–87	88+

Section 6: Safety Habits   My Score:_____

SCORE	1	2	3	4	5	6	7	8	9	10
RATTLE	0–15	16–36	36–54	55–73	74–92	93–111	112–129	130–148	149–168	169+
BEAR	0–19	20–39	40–59	60–78	79–98	99–119	120–139	140–160	161–180	181+
BACKPACK	0–9	10–19	20–31	32–43	44–55	56–66	67–78	79–90	91–102	103+

Overall Score:_____

SCORE	1	2	3	4	5	6	7	8	9	10
RATTLE	0–47	48–93	94–141	142–187	188–236	237–285	286–332	333–380	381–441	442+
BEAR	0–57	58–121	122–185	186–246	247–308	309–372	373–434	435–496	497–561	562+
BACKPACK	0–47	48–101	102–157	158–211	212–265	266–319	320–373	374–426	427–483	484+

Fill in your score for each section, then add them up to get your child's overall score.

SECTION	SCORE
General Health and Medical Conditions	_____
Nutrition	_____
Physical and Mental Exercise	_____
Personal Care	_____
Social and Emotional Health	_____
Safety Habits	_____
OVERALL SCORE	_____

What does your overall score mean?

If you got a 1 or 2

Yikes! At this rate, your child's RealAge, or biological age, could be as much as *8 years older* by the time he's in his 30s. That means his body would be 40 when he's really only 32. And the number of years his RealAge can increase gets larger and larger as he gets older.

There's a lot of work to be done, but just by taking this test you've shown that you're ready. Simple lifestyle changes can significantly improve not only your child's but your whole family's health and make everyone's RealAge younger. Today is the day to begin.

If you got a 3 or 4

Oh my! With your child's current habits, her RealAge, or biological age, could be as much as *4 years older* by the time she's in her 30s. That means her body would be nearly 40 when she's really only 36. And the older she gets, the faster her RealAge can increase.

But I know you can do better. You're already encouraging some healthy habits in your child, and taking this test shows you're ready to do even more. The strategies in the upcoming chapters will help you get rolling.

If you got a 5 or 6

Good going! Given his current habits, your child's RealAge, or biological age, will be just about even with his calendar age when he hits his 30s. But don't stop here!

You're already laying a solid foundation for your child's future health. Now's the time to strengthen it even more. We'll show you how to get started in the pages ahead.

If you got a 7 or 8

Impressive! You clearly know a lot about fostering healthy habits in kids. Your child is lucky to have such a smart role model now, and it will really pay off later. In fact, her RealAge, or biological age, could be as much as *4 years younger* by her early 30s. That means she'll look and feel like she's 30 when she's really 34. And her RealAge can decrease even more as she gets older. Later on, you'll find ways to continue motivating great behavior in your kid.

If you got a 9 or 10

Wow! Take a bow. As an outstanding role model, you're giving your child the greatest gift possible—a strong foundation for a lifetime of healthy habits. Your knowledge and dedication will have a huge impact on his RealAge, or biological age, down the road. It could be as much as *8 years younger* by his 30s. That means he'll look and feel like he's 31 when he's pushing 40.

Where to Go from Here

If you're in the "Wow" group, congratulations. But even if you're at "Yikes" or "Oh my," don't be discouraged. You and your child have so much potential, and today is the day to start tapping it. This book will help you develop a comprehensive program that will make your child safer and healthier today, while providing long-term health benefits for tomorrow. It sounds like a big endeavor—and it is—but we'll break it down into manageable steps, guiding you along the way. Start making a few of them, retake the test in a few months, and watch your score soar!

How to Make Changes That Will Stick

The experts at RealAge long ago dug into the research on how to make successful changes. First, allow a little time—it generally takes ninety days to turn a major change into a true habit.

Second, it helps to realize that forming a good habit—or breaking a bad one—occurs in three stages:

- First, identifying the specific behavior pattern that needs to be changed
- Next, being clear about why changing it is important
- Finally, developing strategies for making the healthy change.

Using these stages, we've developed a framework for building healthy habits in kids. We call it the 4 Is: identify, inform, instruct, and instill.

1. Identify	2. Inform	3. Instruct	4. Instill
Determine the habit that needs to be adopted or modified.	Explain why this habit is vital to health and happiness.	Help your child develop and master the habit.	Reinforce the habit with reminders and support.

The RealAge Healthy Kids Test covers step 1—it *identifies* both good habits and those that need changing. Recheck your scores for each section and then list the ones that need the most improvement.

Ideally, you're striving for a score of 10 in all six areas. Every section of the test has a chapter or two that goes with it, and guides you through steps 2 through 4—*inform, instruct,* and *instill.*

This book is designed to be tailored to fit you and your family's unique needs, so use it in the way that's best for you. For example, if you scored well on the nutrition section, you might skim the chapter on nutrition but focus on the chapters about physical fitness or safety.

Also, because different age groups have such different concerns and issues, sections of some chapters are marked with the rattle, bear, or backpack icons. However, keep in mind that these age ranges, particularly for the rattle and the bear, may overlap since development can vary from child to child.

	If your child is under 2, read the rattle sections first. Then read the bear and backpack sections to see what to expect in the years ahead.
	If your child is 2–9, focus on the sections marked with a bear. Check the backpack sections for what to expect in the years ahead.
	If your child is 10 or older, focus on the sections marked with a backpack.

How Fast Will *Your* Child Change?

Just like adults, some children are more adaptable to transitions than others. For some kids, breaking an old habit or establishing a new one may take fewer than ninety days; for others, it may take longer. Remain active and involved, offering your support and acknowledging the effort that's involved in changing. At times your child may falter—and you may waver, too. But your commitment and positive reinforcement will ultimately help your child succeed—and carry healthy new habits into adulthood.

And although many kids resist changes, almost all kids are good at making them, especially if they have loving support. A basic foundation of security and consistency at home helps kids become more flexible and handle the changes that life inevitably brings.

Your overall goal should be to make sure your children have daily routines and dependable people in their lives. Consistent routines help kids understand what is expected of them, yet still leave room for a range of choices. This familiarity is comforting and allows children to feel as if they have some control over their lives. It's like an internal navigation system—they can find their way around their world without feeling lost or out of control. By the way, it's a good idea to let kids help establish their daily routines—it makes sticking with schedules less a battle of wills.

You'll need to examine your kid's routines from time to time, just to make sure everything is running smoothly:

- Do they seem content with their routines?
- Do they need more downtime?
- Do they have new interests you'd like to encourage?

Good habits are the end product of an ongoing process, one that begins in the first weeks of life and continues through the teen years and beyond. Healthy habits take years of work and upkeep. You'll need to remind yourself time after time not to give in to shortcuts and temptations, just because they're easier at the moment. They won't serve your child down the road: If good habits aren't established, unhealthy bad habits will be formed in their place.

Let's make sure this doesn't happen by getting started on informing, instructing, instilling, and—most important—inspiring.

Chapter 2

EAT UP
Creating Healthy Food Habits That Will Last a Lifetime
(no, they don't have to give up fries forever)

Pediatricians have heard it all. Toddlers who painstakingly find every pea in their meal and drop them off their highchair trays. Five-year-olds who sit on their sandwich and say "all done!" Tweens who use the ol' "under the mashed potatoes" trick . . . as if we didn't do that ourselves. Is it really worth the struggle to get children to eat a balanced diet?

Hm. Well, consider this. Kids who get to eat whatever they want will do just that . . . even if it makes them sick. Even if it makes them grumpy. Or listless. Or out of control. Kids aren't likely to connect a dinner of fries and purple ketchup with not being able to concentrate on homework later on.

But you will.

So how do you improve your child's behavior, mood, and academic performance today—and reduce the likelihood of obesity, high blood pressure, diabetes, or heart disease tomorrow?

You fill your house with a variety of good foods—fruits,

vegetables, whole grains, low-fat dairy products, lean meats, poultry, fish, beans, eggs, and nuts. Then, rather than battling over every Brussels sprout and bean, you get your children involved in planning and preparing meals. For kids, eating dishes they've helped create is completely different from eating foods that are "good for you."

Above all, don't just serve the foods you know your child already likes. It's like school: Your child is constantly exploring new subjects there. You want him to constantly be learning about new foods at home. This will pave the way for a lifetime of better moods and better health.

Dr. Jen's Thirty-Second Energy Quiz

Does your child:

Underperform in school?
Yes ____
No____

Resist playing outside?
Yes____
No____

Become irritable and prone to meltdowns?
Yes____
No____

Appear to be lazy?
Yes____
No____

Show little interest in activities he/she used to enjoy?
Yes____
No____

Have difficulty concentrating for long?
Yes____
No____

If you answered "Yes" to two or more questions, your child may lack the energy to function throughout the day. Good eating habits could help.

Striving for the Perfect Balance

That said, don't worry about the balance of your child's diet in a single meal. Think about it in terms of a week. Focusing on broader patterns is a much more constructive approach.

> **Dr. Jen's Action Step**
>
> Think about your child's nutrient intake over a week, not just one day. When you add it all up, are all the food groups covered? If yes, then you're on the right track. If no, read on for tips on improving your child's diet.

Also, all kids go through stages. At times, they will honestly not be hungry. Usually, this happens in a dormant phase of their growth cycle and it's okay for them not to eat much then. Just brace yourself: The next thing you know, they'll be ravenous and you won't be able to keep enough food in the house.

In addition, kids of all ages tend to hate at least one thing—say, green beans—and devour tons of another, like grapes. Don't worry about a few extremes; if your child's intake over the course of a week, on most weeks, is overall balanced, it's fine.

Portion, Portion, How Big Is a Portion?

How do you know if kids are eating too much? Easy: They gain extra weight. Your pediatrician can help you determine what weight is normal for your child and what's not. Again, depending on growth spurts and activity levels, the amount kids eat can vary a lot. What seems like too much to you might be just what their growing bodies need at the time. If the food is healthy, most kids will eat till they are disinterested or distracted, which usually means they are full. On the other hand, if you're worried that your child isn't eating *enough,* keep in mind that compared with adult servings, a child's serving is pretty small. For instance, a toddler-sized portion may be just a couple of tablespoons.

Start Small

Young children—under age 4—generally eat till they're not hungry, then stop. However, as kids get older, they tend to start ignoring their internal hunger cues and eat according to other influences, such as the amount of food on their plate. Studies show that serving children larger portions encourages them to eat more.

So rather than dishing out a lot of food, start with small servings, and use small, lunch-sized plates rather than dinner plates so meals don't look skimpy. Then, offer seconds if your child is still hungry. One of the keys to maintaining a healthy relationship with food is learning how to gauge internal hunger cues.

Also, serve water with meals, not sugared or carbonated drinks, and encourage kids to take their time when eating. It takes about twenty minutes for the brain to register that the stomach is full, so overeating is frequently the result of eating too fast. Finally, let go of the notion that meals end with dessert, unless it's fruit.

Analyzing Your Answers to the RealAge Healthy Kids Test Nutrition Questions

You probably know all the major players in the nutrition game:

- Grains
- Fruits
- Vegetables
- Dairy products
- Meat/chicken/fish/eggs
- Fats

But do you know how much of each group kids should eat every day? Use the following charts as a guideline, based on their age.

Recommended Daily Food Group Amounts
for Boys and Girls, Ages 2 to 18

Girls Age	Grains	Fruits	Vegetables	Dairy Foods	Meat, Chicken, Fish, Eggs	Fats	Total Daily Calories
2	3 oz.	1 cup	1 cup	2 cups	2 oz.	3 tsp.	1,000
3	4 oz.	1 cup	1½ cups	2 cups	3 oz.	4 tsp.	1,200
4–6	5 oz.	1½ cups	1½ cups	2 cups	4 oz.	4 tsp.	1,400
7–9	5 oz.	1½ cups	2 cups	3 cups	5 oz.	5 tsp.	1,600
10–11	6 oz.	1½ cups	2½ cups	3 cups	5 oz.	5 tsp.	1,800
12–18	6 oz.	2 cups	2½ cups	3 cups	5½ oz.	6 tsp.	2,000

These amounts are based on moderate activity level; to learn more, go to mypyramid.gov.

Boys Age	Grains	Fruits	Vegetables	Dairy Foods	Meat, Chicken, Fish, Eggs	Fats	Total Daily Calories
2	3 oz.	1 cup	1 cup	2 cups	2 oz.	3 tsp.	1,000
3	5 oz.	1½ cups	1½ cups	2 cups	4 oz.	4 tsp.	1,400
4–5	5 oz.	1½ cups	1½ cups	2 cups	4 oz.	4 tsp.	1,400
6–8	5 oz.	1½ cups	2 cups	3 cups	5 oz.	5 tsp.	1,600
9–10	6 oz.	1½ cups	2½ cups	3 cups	5 oz.	5 tsp.	1,800
11	6 oz.	2 cups	2½ cups	3 cups	5½ oz.	6 tsp.	2,000
12–13	7 oz.	2 cups	3 cups	3 cups	6 oz.	6 tsp.	2,200
14	8 oz.	2 cups	3 cups	3 cups	6½ oz.	7 tsp.	2,400
15	9 oz.	2 cups	3½ cups	3 cups	6½ oz.	8 tsp.	2,600
16–18	10 oz.	2½ cups	3½ cups	3 cups	7 oz.	8 tsp.	2,800

These amounts are based on moderate activity level; to learn more, go to mypyramid.gov.

Unfortunately, while kids today are getting enough calories—often more than enough—too few of these calories are coming from nutritionally sound sources. A recent study of 2- to 11-year-olds showed that about one-third of them were not meeting the daily requirements for fruits, grains, meats, dairy products, and vegetables. Perhaps most surprising, 16 percent did not meet any of the recommendations at all! So, where are kids' calories coming from? You guessed it: fats and sugars—two things that should be playing minor roles in their diets.

Filling up on "junk," such as chips, cookies, and soft drinks, usually means that protein, fiber, healthy fats, and essential vitamins and minerals get pushed out. The result over time: A greater risk for a number of health problems, including obesity, heart disease, and diabetes, just to name a few.

That's not to say that fat should be eliminated from a child's diet. Actually, during the early childhood years, kids need dietary fat for proper growth and neurological development (see the charts on page 38 for specific amounts). Fat also helps the body absorb certain nutrients and is necessary for maintaining energy levels. But fat should come from nutritious foods such as nuts, avocados, olive and vegetable oils, and low-fat dairy products (yogurt, cheese, and milk). Until the age of 2, children need whole-fat dairy products; after that, switching to lower-fat options is generally acceptable. Fat should make up a little less than a third of your child's diet. However, because individual needs vary, discuss this with your child's pediatrician.

Diversifying Your Child's Food Portfolio

Food is good medicine; each group contains hundreds of unique and powerful substances that promote good health.

While getting an appropriate amount of each major kind of food every day is a good start, in order to make your child's diet really work, you need to tap the wide range of nutrient-rich foods *within* each group.

Take It Slow

To introduce more foods into a kid's diet, don't try to revamp the family's eating habits overnight. First tackle the excesses and then focus on the deficiencies. Modest changes are more likely to add up to positive, lifelong eating habits.

Try to slowly expand the menu by focusing on what I call the three Ts: tint (color), texture, and taste. You can't go wrong if you have a good variety of these on the plate. Here's why:

Tint—The more colorful the mix of food on the plate, the greater the nutritional payoff. Richly colored fruits and veggies—bright berries, sunny tangerines, emerald spinach, red bell peppers—contain important protective phytochemicals and antioxidants that help prevent disease and preserve health in many ways. They also can help cool inflammatory activity in the body that, among other things, contributes to heart and blood vessel disease.

Allow a little more time than usual on your next grocery run. When you hit the produce aisle, focus more on the colors than on specific foods. Use this grocery list to help you explore.

How to Keep Your Family's Diet Colorful

Bring this to the store and pick up at least 2 items from each color every week!*				
RED	**WHITE-GREEN**	**BLUE-PURPLE**	**YELLOW-ORANGE**	**YELLOW-GREEN**
__tomatoes	__leeks	__blackberries	__apricots	__bananas
__watermelon	__garlic	__blueberries	__cantaloupe	__avocados
__cherries	__chives	__black currants	__grapefruit	__green apples
__cranberries	__brown pears	__dried plums	__lemons	__green grapes
__strawberries	__dates	__elderberries	__mangoes	__honeydew
__raspberries	__cauliflower	__purple figs	__nectarines	melon
__pomegranates	__ginger	__red grapes	__oranges	__kiwifruit
__pink grapefruit	__mushrooms	__plums	__papayas	__limes
__beets	__onions	__raisins	__peaches	__green pears
__red peppers	__parsnips	__red cabbage	__persimmons	__artichokes
__radishes	__shallots	__eggplant	__pineapple	__arugula
__radicchio	__scallions	__purple peppers	__tangerines	__asparagus
__red potatoes	__turnips		__squash	__broccoli
__red apples			__carrots	__Brussels sprouts
__rhubarb			__yellow peppers	__cabbage
			__pumpkin	__celery
			__rutabagas	__cucumbers
			__sweet potatoes	__endive
				__leafy greens
				__green onions
				__okra
				__peas
				__green peppers
				__snow peas
				__sugar snap peas
				__spinach
				__watercress
				__zucchini
*Eat edible peels whenever possible—they're rich in fiber and nutrients. Wash them thoroughly first.				

Texture—Keep things crunchy with veggies, whole grains, seeds, and nuts. All are nutritional powerhouses and many are filled with insoluble fiber, which helps ward off type 2 diabetes and works to keep your child's colon healthy by helping intestinal function. Insoluble fiber is mainly found in whole grains like oats, barley, brown rice, whole-wheat breads and pasta, and whole-grain breakfast cereals, but veggies like carrots, zucchini, celery, Brussels sprouts, cabbage, and cauliflower are packed with it, too. Sunflower, sesame, and pumpkin seeds are healthy sources of vitamins, minerals, protein, amino acids, and good (unsaturated) fats, so sprinkle them on main dishes, salads, and sandwiches. The same goes for nuts such as cashews, almonds, walnuts, pecans, and pine nuts.

Taste—Introduce your child to new flavors by cooking with different herbs, spices, and sauces. Depending on how adventuresome your kid is, gradually try out the combinations suggested in the chart below. With stronger flavors (ginger, dill, horseradish), use a light hand at first. Some will fly, some won't—for now—but every bit of progress counts.

VEGETABLE FLAVOR BOOSTERS	ENTRÉE TASTE TURN-ONS
• **Tomatoes:** Basil, oregano, marjoram	• **Chicken:** Lemon juice, garlic, paprika, coriander, cumin
• **Carrots:** Orange juice, coriander, chives	• **Pork:** Orange juice, garlic, ginger, green onions
• **Peas:** Parsley, onions, mint	• **Beef:** Black pepper, ginger, horseradish, mustard
• **Green beans:** Lemon juice, mustard seeds	• **Fish:** Lemon juice, paprika, parsley, dill, black pepper
• **Potatoes:** Chives, green onions, dill, parsley, turmeric	

Applying this 3-Ts strategy to family meals will help ensure that your child has the right balance of calories, proteins, minerals, and vitamins—not only for healthy physical growth but also for proper brain development, weight control, disease prevention, and more.

Okay, let's move on to specific food habits, starting with meal number one: breakfast.

On most weeks, how many times per week does your child eat breakfast?

How many times have you heard, "breakfast is the most important meal of the day"? Well, it bears repeating. A morning meal makes everything better—better energy, better concentration, better problem-solving skills, and better eye–hand coordination. That means better performance in school and a better appreciation and love for learning.

What's more, breakfast eaters tend to be healthier eaters overall, and these eating patterns usually continue into adulthood, helping people maintain a healthy weight and avoid heart disease and other serious health problems in the years ahead.

RealAge Projection: **Getting into the habit of eating breakfast every day will benefit kids for years to come. If they keep this habit up into adulthood, they'll stay 39 when they should be turning 40.**

Let's Do Breakfast

Granted, it's not always an easy task. Mornings are usually pretty hectic and getting a kid to eat more than a few bites before rushing to play or catch the bus is a challenge. But a few bites are better than nothing and you can work up from there.

TOP 5 REASONS WHY BREAKFAST IS A MUST	TOP 5 EXCUSES FOR SKIPPING BREAKFAST
Kids who eat breakfast . . . • Do better in school. • Have better focus and concentration. • Have fewer behavioral problems. • Are more likely to meet their nutritional needs. • Have an easier time staying at a healthy weight.	• "But Mom, I ate all of my dinner last night!" • "I'm gonna miss the bus!" • "That cereal doesn't snap-crackle-pop!" • "I already brushed my teeth!" • "I'm not hungry!" Don't give in to kids' woeful pleas! Make breakfast a morning ritual for you both.

Mornings at my house are usually like a game of beat the clock, so I try to organize what I can the night before, enlisting the help of my kids. We pick out clothes, plan lunches, and place backpacks next to the front door so that in the morning, breakfast can be a priority.

Other families set fruit, cereal, and dishes on the table and put perishable foods on a refrigerator tray, ready to whisk to the table in the morning.

If you can't make the morning meal happen at home, send the kids off with healthy on-the-go breakfasts to eat on the way to school or when they arrive. Have them help you fill plastic zipper bags with things like nuts, raisins, and other dried fruits; orange slices; low-fat granola; hard-boiled eggs; cheese and crackers; sliced apple sandwich "cookies" filled with peanut butter; or other nutritious, portable options that they can munch on.

Nowadays more and more schools are providing breakfast

in an effort to boost academic performance and attendance and reduce behavior problems. These programs appear to be working— many schools report significant improvements, academically and socially.

So, what does your child typically eat for breakfast?
It doesn't have to be fancy. In fact, there's growing evidence that a bowl of good old-fashioned oatmeal may be ideal. Several recent studies have shown that when kids eat oatmeal for breakfast— versus cold cereal or no breakfast at all—they have better memory and attention, skills that come in handy when studying subjects like math and geography. Scientists think this effect is linked to whole-grain oatmeal's high-fiber, high-protein content. Because whole grains digest slowly, they supply the brain with a steady stream of energy.

Beat Breakfast Boredom

Stumped for some new breakfasts to get your kids going? Try some of these variations on the morning meal:

Easy Smoothies: Combine 2 frozen bananas, 1 cup of strawberries, 1 cup low-fat vanilla yogurt, and ¾ cup juice in a blender. Makes 2 servings.

Oatmeal Cookie Pancakes: To your regular pancake batter, add oats, raisins, cinnamon, chopped walnuts, and a bit of brown sugar. Then pour into fun shapes like Mickey Mouse. Make the batter the night before and keep it in the fridge to beat the morning rush.

Breakfast Tacos: Spoon scrambled eggs into warm corn tortillas, top with shredded cheese, a dollop of low-fat yogurt or sour cream, and salsa.

Open-face Sandwiches: Spread whole-grain toast with peanut butter and whole-fruit puree, or even guacamole and salsa for adventurous teens.

Whether your child's favorite cereal is hot or cold, always check the nutrition label for fiber, protein, and sugar content per serving. At breakfast, you want to get plenty of fiber and protein into kids because it will keep them feeling full and energized until lunch. For the same reason, aim to keep sugar to a minimum;

otherwise, it can send a kid's energy soaring up, then tumbling down before the morning's half over. In fact, sugar of any kind should not be among the first three ingredients on the label.

What should be there:

- Fiber—at least 3 grams per serving; add a fistful of fresh fruit, raisins, dried cranberries, almonds, pecans, sunflower seeds, ground flax seed, or wheat germ, to bring the total to 6 grams
- Protein—at least 3 grams per serving
- Sugar—no more than 5 grams per serving

Hint: If your child's favorite cereal is low on fiber, try mixing it with another cereal that's high in fiber.

The other morning nutrient you need to focus on is fat—specifically, the healthy polyunsaturated fatty acids (PUFAs) that are high in omega-3s. Why? A recent study found that kids who eat more of these fats do better on short-term memory tests than kids who eat more saturated fat (the bad, artery-clogging kind found in butter, among other things). One of the easiest ways to get good omega-3 fats into your kids is to sprinkle walnuts or almonds on their cereal. You can also make breakfast from omega-3–enriched eggs, which are now widely available, and spread canola oil (another good source) instead of butter on their whole-grain toast. A bit of healthy fat will help your child feel fuller for longer, and also helps her body better absorb other nutrients from the meal.

If your child prefers breakfast bars, be sure to read labels the

Fiber Rule of Thumb

Here's an easy way to estimate how many grams a day growing kids need: **Take their age and add 5 to 10 grams of fiber to it.** That's the minimum range, and some experts think kids' fiber intake should be much higher, which is one reason high-fiber whole-grain cereals and breads are so important.

same way you would cereal labels, noting fat, fiber, protein, and sugar content. Many bars tend to skimp on fiber and bulk up on sugar. It's best if sugar or corn syrup is not among the first three ingredients in breakfast foods.

RealAge Projection: **Kids who get into the habit of eating fiber-rich foods now are likely to stick with this healthy habit as adults. And if they do—getting 25 grams of fiber a day as an adult—by age 32, their RealAge could actually be only 29.**

Give Breakfast a Boost

Eggs are another breakfast food that can help make kids feel full until lunchtime. Thanks to what turned out to be a bad cholesterol rap, people avoided eggs for years. But eggs have always been a good source of nutrients and protein and a major medical study has cleared them of upping heart attack and stroke risk.

If your family is hooked on breakfast meats, opt for leaner ones, such as Canadian bacon, and/or limit them to once a week. Traditional breakfast meats tend to be high in saturated fat and/or sodium. You also can substitute chicken, turkey, or soy-based bacon and sausage. There are several good choices on the market, but check the labels for fat and sodium content; some brands can be high.

If pancakes or waffles are a family tradition, look for buckwheat mixes or add several tablespoons of bran to the batter to boost the fiber content. Also, top hotcakes with fresh fruit purees, yogurt, or a handful of berries instead of syrup and butter.

Washing breakfast down with milk is a good choice for all age groups (though make it low-fat after age 2), and, while it shouldn't replace fresh fruit, 4 to 8 ounces of 100 percent juice per day is fine, too. (Read more about juice on page 51.)

Let's talk about beverages next. What does your child drink most often?

Liquids do more than just quench kids' thirst. Beverages replace the liquid their bodies lose through activity and normal body function and, when chosen wisely, can also provide a nutritional boost.

So make sure your child's beverages count.

Plain old water is best for keeping small bodies hydrated and functioning at their best, but other drinks, such as low-fat milk and 100 percent juice, can be a good way to fill in nutritional holes. Steering kids toward these beverages and away from sugar- or caffeine-filled drinks can help them maintain a healthy weight and healthy smile for years to come.

Is Organic Milk Healthier?

Milk production has changed quite a bit in the past few decades, as "factory farming"—in which cows are crammed into giant feedlots—has almost wiped out the natural system of grazing cows in pastures. Although factory farming increases milk output, the milk is somewhat less nutritious. Organic milk that comes from grass-fed cows (not all of it does) may be a healthier choice than regular commercial milk. But expect to pay more.

Babies and Milk

If you're not able to breastfeed for the entire first year of your baby's life, as the American Academy of Pediatrics recommends, be assured that even nursing for a few weeks gives your newborn some nutritional and immune-system benefits. If you stop breastfeeding before one year, switch to iron-fortified formula, not cow's milk. Your pediatrician can guide you in selecting one that is just right for your baby.

Optimize Bone Health Early

Think of bone as a savings account; kids' bodies constantly make *deposits* and *withdrawals* of bone tissue. During childhood and adolescence, more bone is deposited than withdrawn as the skeleton grows in both size and density. A diet rich in calcium and other minerals keeps withdrawals, or bone loss, to a minimum. Kids with the highest peak bone mass after adolescence have the greatest advantage in terms of future bone health. So optimizing bone health early in life is crucial in preventing future fractures and osteoporosis. Soda, alcohol, high caffeine consumption, certain medications, antacids that contain aluminum, calorie restriction, and a lack of exercise are some common causes of low bone density.

If your child doesn't drink milk or eat any other high-calcium foods, such as yogurt, cheese, or calcium-fortified orange juice, then taking a multivitamin containing vitamin D *and* a calcium supplement is essential.

American Academy of Pediatrics Recommendations on Calcium Intake	
Age	**Calcium**
1–3 years	500 mg per day (the equivalent of about 2 one-cup servings of milk)
4–8 years	800 mg per day (the equivalent of about 3 one-cup servings of low-fat milk)
9–18 years	1,300 mg per day (the equivalent of about 4 one-cup servings of low-fat milk)

RealAge Projection: If kids get into the habit of eating calcium-rich foods now, they're likely to stick with this habit as adults. And by getting 400 IU of vitamin D and 1,200 milligrams of calcium in their adult diet, they could look and feel as much as 1.3 years younger at age 35.

When Bone Density Gets Low

Rachel, an active, sports-minded 16-year-old, came to see me because she injured her wrist while playing volleyball for her high school team. It turned out to be a wrist fracture, her third fracture in three years. With a little probing, I discovered that Rachel wasn't drinking milk because she "didn't like the taste." So, instead she drank a lot of sodas, which contain caffeine and phosphorous, both substances that leech out calcium. Worse, she also admitted to me that she'd been smoking—another bone weakener. Although Rachel intentionally ate a lot of lean protein for muscle growth, she avoided cheese and other dairy products, afraid that they would make her gain weight.

A bone-density scan revealed what I feared: Rachel's bone density was low—she even showed early signs of osteoporosis. Some simple changes to her diet would help Rachel reverse the damage, strengthen her bones, and avoid the fractures that are common in kids who don't get enough calcium—which includes

---

Sunscreen, Milk, and Vitamin D Deficiency

Sunlight makes skin produce vitamin D. So during winter's short, cloudy, indoor days, everyone runs some risk of becoming deficient in this vitamin. Kids with darker skin or who live in northern areas without much sun are most at risk. In addition, in nice weather kids today often leave the house wearing sunscreen. That's a good thing in terms of skin cancer. But it limits the benefit of brief exposure to the sun. So what do I recommend?

Milk and cereal for breakfast.

Most milk is fortified with vitamin D, as are many breakfast cereals. Vitamin D helps the body absorb calcium and works with calcium to strengthen bones. The recommended dose of vitamin D is 200 IUs per day, the amount in 2 cups of fortified milk.

If you have a child who can't or won't drink milk, the best alternative may be a multivitamin.

most older children and adolescents in the United States. Only 10 percent of adolescent girls get the recommended 1,300 mg of calcium per day. So discourage soft drinks and get more calcium into kids by giving them calcium-enriched orange juice and breakfast smoothies. (Throw some berries and bananas into these too. Take every opportunity to include fruits and veggies in your child's diet.)

Juice Facts

Since few children consistently meet the recommended intake of fruits and vegetables, sipping a moderate amount of 100 percent juice is one way to fill in some of their nutrient gaps. Juice is a great source of vitamin C and is often fortified with calcium. And because it's on the sweet side, even the pickiest of children enjoy it. What's more, several products now contain both fruit and vegetable juice, including Vruit, Odwalla, V8 V.Fusion, and Juice Plus, among others.

The key with juice is to sip, not guzzle. Be wary of allowing your child to fill up on juice—there may not be room left for the other foods needed for a well-balanced diet. Also, juices often are high in simple sugars and calories, which promote tooth decay and weight gain. They also lack the fiber and full nutritional punch of whole fruits and vegetables, so they're not a full replacement for these foods. For example, whole apples are high in protective phytochemicals that may help reduce the risk of certain types of cancer, asthma, diabetes, and cardiovascular disease. Apple juice isn't.

Actually, I recommend no juice at all until age 1—the age when most kids can start drinking juice from a cup rather than a bottle—to reduce tooth decay. After age 2, limit daily intake to 4–6 ounces of 100 percent juice. Many parents dilute juice with water to make it last throughout the day and reduce the amount of sugar their child consumes. However, I'd rather a child just drink the juice all at once and then drink water the rest of the day. Not only is this much healthier for teeth but most of my patients' parents who follow this advice report that their children now pick water as their first choice of drink.

Replace Lost Fluids

The importance of kids staying hydrated during intense physical activity is often overlooked. The more vigorous the activity, or the warmer the weather, the more critical it is for them to take in enough fluids. Talk with kids about how often and how much they should be drinking.

This will vary from child to child, so teach kids to pay attention to signs that they may be getting a little dehydrated, such as their lips being dry or their mouth feeling gummy or sticky. With increased dehydration comes shakiness, headaches, and stomachaches.

Water is the best choice for overall hydration, unless you've got a superactive kid. Your child may prefer sports drinks like Gatorade or Propel, but some sports drinks contain caffeine and many have high-fructose corn syrup—which will add to your kid's daily calorie intake and has some worrisome side effects (see page 53).

Sweet Sipping

Many experts partly blame the dramatic increase in childhood obesity on the overconsumption of sweetened soft drinks such as soda, iced tea, punch, and artificially flavored fruit beverages. A single 12-ounce can of these has as much as 13 teaspoons of sugar in the form of high-fructose corn syrup (HFCS). This thick liquid is made from cornstarch and, unlike other sweeteners, it disrupts the body's production of certain hormones that help regulate appetite and fat storage. As a result, some nutrition experts believe that HFCS-sweetened beverages throw off the body's normal weight-regulating mechanisms. That means kids get a bunch of empty calories that leave their bodies craving even more calories. A recent study revealed that drinking one can of sugary soda a day increases their risk of becoming obese by 60 percent!

As for young teeth, sodas are doubly destructive because their sugar promotes decay, while their acidity destroys protective enamel—even in sugar-free sodas. In addition, adolescents, who need more than double the calcium of young children, are increasingly choosing soda over milk, which puts their bone development and overall healthy growth in jeopardy.

Now, consider a typical week. Does your child get enough vegetables and fruits in his/her diet?
For many parents, getting their children to eat the recommended five-or-more-a-day seems like an impossible dream. But given all the power these foods pack, it's a dream worth pursuing.

> *RealAge Projection:* Getting kids in the habit of eating plenty of fruits and vegetables will benefit them for years to come . . . but only if they keep it up throughout childhood and into adulthood. If they do, their RealAge could be 36 when their birthday cards say "Happy 40th!"

Get a handle on how many servings of fruit and veggies your child really needs.

- Ages 6 months to 6 years: about five servings—two of fruit, three of vegetables.
- Older children and teen girls: about seven servings—three of fruit, four of vegetables.
- Teen boys: about nine servings—four of fruit, five of vegetables.

Getting five to nine servings of fruit and vegetables each day may sound like a lot of produce, but serving sizes may be smaller than you think. For a child under 2 years, a serving is only about 1 ounce, or about 2 tablespoons. For children over 2, a serving is any of the following:

- 1 medium-sized fruit
- ½ cup raw, cooked, frozen, or canned fruits or vegetables (cherry tomatoes, pea pods, mandarin oranges)
- ¼ cup dried fruit (raisins, figs, cherries, cranberries)
- 1 cup raw, leafy vegetables (spinach, lettuce, bok choy)
- ½ cup cooked, canned, or frozen legumes (beans, corn, peas)
- ¾ cup 100 percent fruit or vegetable juice
- 1 cup vegetable soup

These can be spread out through the day. For example, for lunch serve toddlers ¼ cup of vegetables, or half a medium-sized piece of fresh fruit; then give them the rest of the fruit for a snack and two ¼-cup servings of veggies at dinner. A good rule of thumb is to make fruits and veggies part of every meal.

While getting some children to eat fruits and vegetables can be difficult, don't let it turn into a battle. Try this technique: When a new food is on the dinner plate, I ask my kids to taste it; if they don't like it, I don't give them a hard time about it. I prepare it again, about a week later. It gives them another chance to try it, and sometimes they actually like it. In fact, about half the time, they like it the first time! Not bad odds at all.

Also, try adapting a strategy from grocery stores: Put the food you want to "move" where your "customers" can't miss it. Always keep fresh fruit on the counter where it's easy to grab and place veggies at the front and center of the refrigerator. That way when kids get the urge to munch, they'll be more likely to reach for a peach or some pea pods and carrots, especially if they are already cut up. If you're pressed for time, buy packaged, ready-to-go fruits and veggies. It might cost more, but it's cheaper than a box of cookies—or filling a cavity.

When kids are young, try making weekly fruit and vegetable charts together, and have your child place a star for each vegetable or fruit eaten. Hang it on the refrigerator for inspiration.

 ### Start Early

As with other healthy habits, it's much easier if you start when kids are young. At about 6 months, it's time to begin leading babies into the world of solid foods. Since babies burn through the bulk of the iron reserves that they're born with by 6 months, iron-fortified infant cereal is usually recommended as the first food. But fruits and vegetables can be introduced soon afterward.

Babies have preferences, just like you do. Some will gobble up squash and reject applesauce. Or vice versa. Try not to be rigid about your expectations. Introduce a broad range of foods and allow your baby to embrace or reject anything. But be persistent. Reoffer foods that your baby initially refused. After the fifteenth try, she may surprise you and discover a new favorite.

Use the guide below as a general rule to figure out what and how much to give your baby. Or, look for cues that your baby is full. If she becomes disinterested, looks away, or shakes her head no, it usually means she's had enough. And the more solid food she eats, the less formula or breast milk she'll want.

Food	Times Daily	Amount
Baby cereal (rice, oat, barley)	1–2	1–4 tbsp.
Fruit (applesauce, bananas, peaches, pears)	2	2–3 tbsp.
Vegetables (squash, carrots, green beans, peas)	2	2–3 tbsp.
Fruit juice (best after 2 years of age)	1	3 oz.

  Getting a Late Start?

If you didn't get your baby started early on fruits and vegetables, be prepared to get creative—even downright sneaky if necessary. Whatever you do, don't preach. Telling a child "It's good for you!" is just an invitation to resist.

Below are a few suggestions for slipping these important foods into your child's diet.

- **Grate 'em up**—Add finely chopped vegetables to soups, stews, meatballs, meatloaf, and spaghetti sauce. They can't pick out what they can't see.
- **Drop 'em in**—Add bananas or dried fruit to cereal or pancakes.
- **Cover 'em up**—Serve vegetables with cheese sauce or yogurt dips (Bonus: source of calcium).
- **Uncook 'em**—Serve both raw and cooked vegetables. A child might love raw cauliflower but loathe it cooked.

- **Bean 'em up**—Legumes count as vegetables. Try serving mild-tasting peas and beans such as baby lima beans, chickpeas, great northern (white) beans, pinto beans, lentils, and edamame. Some will get accepted.
- **Carve 'em up**—Make it fun! Create food faces with cut-up vegetables; make a colorful swirl with sliced fruit.
- **Pair 'em**—Pair favorite foods with more unfamiliar fruits and vegetables, like oranges and kiwis, or potatoes and artichokes.

Avoiding Allergies

Parents have long been advised to avoid introducing certain foods—dairy products, wheat, and spices, for example—before a specific age. These foods do seem to cause an allergic response in some children. So it's wise to be cautious about the timing of new foods, especially if you, your partner, or a sibling has ever had an unfavorable food reaction.

With all kids I suggest introducing new foods slowly, beginning with single-ingredient foods and spacing the addition of each new food at least three or four days apart. With this approach, you can watch for any adverse reactions. If none appear, continue on. If your child does have an adverse reaction, eliminate the food and talk with your pediatrician.

For families with a history of food allergies, hold off on introducing solids until kids are at least 6 months old. After that, start off with an iron-fortified rice or oat cereal (wait on wheat cereals until 12 months). Then, gradually add vegetables over the next few weeks, but avoid beans, peas, and other legumes for a month or two. Next, add fruits (except berries and citrus) but avoid all dairy products until at least age 1. At 8 months, add meat and poultry. At age 1, add citrus and dairy foods but avoid eggs and berries until age 2, and avoid fish, shellfish, and nuts until at least age 3.

For kids without any family history of food allergies or sensitivities, you can start citrus, berries, and eggs at age 1 and shellfish and nuts at 2. Wheat, soy, and dairy products are usually fine after 6 months.

Ready for snack time? What are typical snacks for your child?

Somewhere along the line, snacks got a bad rap. Perhaps it was the constant warning, "No snacking between meals, you'll spoil your dinner!" Certainly, munching on too many cookies can cause kids to lose their appetite for meals.

However, when chosen wisely, snacks provide another opportunity for kids to get the nutrients they need. Young kids need smaller portions of food more often since their stomachs are pretty small. The trick is to make sure that snacks pack as much nutritional punch and fiber as possible without a lot of saturated fat and calories.

Small snacks also can be an effective way to prevent overeating; they stave off excessive hunger, so kids don't become ravenous and reach for junk food. On the other hand, children should not be snacking so much that they're not hungry for meals. Establishing set snack times will also help fight emotional eating—snacking because of boredom or stress.

True Parenting Story: The Insatiable Snacker

At 5 years old, Megan was a grazer. She'd routinely leave half of her breakfast uneaten, claiming to be full, then ask for a snack thirty minutes later. I thought it was okay because I tried to keep the snacks healthy—string cheese and pretzels, for example. But as she got used to grazing throughout the day, she rarely ate more than a couple of bites at regular meals. I was frustrated at the waste of food, but I didn't want to deny her a snack if she was really hungry.

At Megan's annual checkup, I asked for some advice. Dr. Jen told me that kids need to snack, but that snacks shouldn't be a substitute for meals. She recommended trying a midmorning and a midafternoon snack, and though I was a bit skeptical, I agreed.

The first day wasn't easy. Megan refused to eat her eggs and toast, so I told her she could stop eating, but I would save it for later, when she got hungry. Sure enough, half an hour later, Megan came to me, begging for a snack. When I reheated breakfast for her, she whined, "No, I want a snack!"

"No snacks unless you eat breakfast." I held firm. She reluctantly ate a few more bites. At 10 a.m., I put out a plate of sliced apples and a graham cracker with peanut butter. "Okay, snack time. This is it until lunch." Megan ate up happily, but soon wanted more to nosh on, and lunch was still an hour away. The hardest part for me was saying no. But when Megan ate most of her turkey sandwich and fruit at lunch, I could see that the schedule was working.

Now, Megan has a snack around 10 a.m. and another around 3 p.m. While she still doesn't clean her plate at meals, I know she's learning better eating habits. I am too.

—LINDA, NEW YORK, NY

Again, think about placement. Make it as easy as possible for your child to reach for that cut-up fruit and yogurt instead of chocolate-chip cookies. If healthy snacks are more convenient, you'll encourage healthy snacking habits.

Snack Attack Fun

These easy-to-whip-up snacks are sure to be a hit with kids of any age:

Creepy-Crawly Crackers: Spread peanut butter between two round wheat crackers, add pretzel sticks for legs and raisins for eyes, and you've got one fun, spidery snack.

A Feast for Giants: Broccoli "trees" are much more fun when you can dunk them in salsa or a yogurt-based dip. Mix up 8 oz. plain yogurt with some chopped fresh dill, a little Dijon mustard, and a dash of soy sauce. Try dunking carrot "logs," bell pepper strip "canoes," cherry tomato "boulders," and cucumber slice "bridges."

Graham sandwiches: Here's a delicious cheesecake-like treat when your child wants something sweet. Spread half a graham cracker with cream cheese, a little raspberry jam, and top with the other cracker half. Yummy!

In a crunch, prepackaged healthy choices are fig bars, trail mix, and single-serving packets of whole-grain cereal.

Bad Disguised as Good

So you're convinced that snacks can be part of a healthy diet. With that in mind, you vow to buy all the "reduced-fat," "no-fat," "low carb," "less sugar," and "all natural" snacks you can find. Hold on a minute. Turn the package over and read the ingredients label.

The ingredients are listed in descending order, by weight. That means the first ingredients play a starring role in the snack you choose for your child. If flour is listed, look for whole grains. They offer many health benefits, including complex carbohydrates, which are healthier because they take longer to digest and help control blood sugar levels.

Be aware that just because something lists "wheat" flour doesn't mean that it's whole wheat. And enriched flour is refined flour that has nutrients added back in. Why take them out in the first place?

Stay away from foods that contain trans fats, which are also listed as hydrogenated or partially hydrogenated oil. Cookies, crackers, icing, potato chips, margarine, and microwave popcorn often contain these fats.

Trans fats are made using a process called hydrogenation that turns unsaturated fats into highly stable saturated fats that resist turning rancid. About twenty years ago, manufacturers began putting trans fats into processed foods to extend their shelf life. However, it turned out that these man-made fats are much riskier than any natural fat, even the saturated fats found in butter, beef, and pork. Several studies have found that trans fats raise the risk of heart disease, increase total cholesterol, and reduce healthy HDL good cholesterol.

> **Whole Grain Quick Tips**
>
> Here's how to incorporate more whole grains and bran into your family's diet:
>
> - Serve whole-grain breakfast cereals such as bran flakes, shredded wheat, oatmeal, or any of the growing number of other whole-grain cereals.
> - Always make toast and sandwiches with whole-grain breads.
> - Cook soup and chili with barley.
> - Serve brown rice, whole-wheat pasta, and whole-wheat couscous instead of white rice and white noodles.

But don't avoid all fat. Just concentrate on the heart-healthy fats found in plant-based foods—nuts, avocados, olive oil, flaxseed and sesame oils, and more.

RealAge Projection: **Kids who develop a taste for foods filled with saturated and trans fats when they're young are likely to keep craving them as they get older. And if bad fats are a regular part of their adult diet, their RealAge** could be more like 35 when they're only 32, due to the damaging effects on arteries and waistlines.

Smart snack choices should give your child's concentration and energy levels a healthy boost. So . . .

Try some of these tasty, and healthy, snacks:

- Trail mix made with whole-grain cereal, peanuts, raisins, and mini dark chocolate chips
- Nachos made with baked corn chips, fat-free refried black beans, shredded chicken, low-fat cheddar cheese, and grated carrots

WHEN KIDS SAY, "I WANT . . ."	ANSWER, "HOW ABOUT . . ."
Frito-Lay *Doritos*	Frito-Lay *Multigrain Tostitos* (whole grains)
McDonald's *Chicken McNuggets*	Morningstar Farms *Buffalo Wings* (no trans fats)
	Perdue *Chicken Breast Nuggets* (no trans fats)
Kellogg's *Pop-Tarts*	Amy's *Toaster Pops* (much less fat and sugar; no trans fats)
Oscar Mayer *Turkey & Cheddar Lunchables*	Nabisco *Triscuits,* low-fat cheese, and Healthy Choice turkey breast slices (whole grains, much less fat and cholesterol)
Girl Scouts *Thin Mints*	Newman's Own Organics *Newman-O's Mint Crème Cookies* (much less saturated fat)
Burger King *Whopper with cheese*	Wendy's Jr. Cheeseburger Deluxe (less than half the fat, calories, cholesterol; almost no trans fats)
All-beef hot dog	Lightlife soy *Smart Dog* (no fat, half the sodium)
French fries	Homemade oven fries—baked, lightly coated with heart-healthy olive oil (half the calories, one quarter the fat)

- Turkey-tortilla roll-ups moistened with low-fat cream cheese, chopped celery, and red pepper
- Whole-wheat waffle topped with peanut butter, whole-fruit spread, or yogurt and berries
- Cherry tomatoes filled with tuna salad or cottage cheese

How many sweets does your child eat throughout the day? Children seem to have a natural inclination toward sweets. And as they grow, so does their sweet tooth.

Although totally restricting processed sweets may be the healthiest option, it might not be the smartest one. Studies have found that exerting too much diet control can backfire—kids who aren't allowed any treats tend to overindulge at the first chance or obsess about forbidden foods. So allow a couple of cookies after dinner once or twice a week and chocolate cake on birthdays. After all, it's not the occasional sugar-filled treat that's detrimental, it's a steady diet of sweets.

Some healthy dessert alternatives for every day are bowls of berries, frozen juice pops, yogurt, or a whole-grain banana muffin. And have you heard? Although it may seem too good to be true, research has shown that dark, cocoa-rich chocolate is also rich in the same protective antioxidants found in apples and grapes.

Not white chocolate. Not milk chocolate. Only rich, dark chocolate containing a minimum of 70 percent cocoa solids. It might taste a bit bitter to kids, but give it a try with some fruit, especially pears or

Liven Up Lunches

If your child is tired of the same-old-same-old, try some of these tips to make lunch more interesting:

Change up the bread: How about low-fat cream cheese with apple slices on cinnamon raisin bread? Or turkey and cranberry sauce on rye?

Have fun with shapes: Use large cookie cutters to make ghost-shaped sandwiches at Halloween, or snowmen in December.

oranges. If it goes over, having one- to two-ounce portions of dark chocolate a few times a week is another healthy way to satisfy a sweet tooth. You can even throw it in as a lunch treat.

> *RealAge Projection:* Getting into the habit of enjoying antioxidant-rich foods like sweet cherries, plums, pecans, and dark chocolate will benefit kids for years to come. If they keep it up throughout childhood and into adulthood, they'll look and feel like they're in their early 40s when they're really 50.

Does your child eat well-balanced, homemade lunches or school lunches?

A lot of parents I talk to would rather give their kids a couple of dollars for a cafeteria lunch than make a brown-bag lunch. The trouble is that school meals tend to sabotage children's eating habits.

Most school cafeterias still serve prepackaged, highly processed foods instead of whole grains, fresh fruits, and vegetables. In addition, you have no way of knowing if your child is skipping the entrée and just eating cheese puffs and cookies. If junk food is available, kids will buy it. Studies show a direct link between the availability of junk food at school and a higher calorie and fat intake during school hours.

With a little planning, it is possible for your child to get a nutritious cafeteria lunch. Make a weekly date to review the school lunch menu together. Discuss what is offered and decide together what's best. It's a great opportunity to work through how to make healthy and tasty choices.

In general, however, bagged lunches are the best way to make sure your child eats healthy foods at school.

To see what they *are* and *are not* eating, ask younger kids to put their leftovers back into their lunch box, so you can see whether they ate that bag of baby carrots or the string cheese. It's a good way to judge what works at lunchtime and what doesn't and talk about options. Also, getting kids involved in making their own healthy lunch the night before increases the odds that they'll actually eat it!

A word about cold cuts: You may find that your child wants to pack a bologna sandwich every day. Having one occasionally is fine, but processed meats are often high in saturated fat, sodium, and preservatives, and shouldn't be daily fare. Solution: Most grocery stores carry not only fresh turkey meat but also a variety of soy- and vegetable-based "deli meat" alternatives. Try them. You—and your kids—may be surprised by how good many brands are.

As far as meats and poultry go, which types does your child eat fairly regularly?

Beef, pork, lamb, and poultry have long been a staple of family dinners. All provide complete protein, which means they contain the nine essential amino acids the body can't make on its own. These amino acids help build muscle cells, immune cells, blood cells, enzymes, and other structures.

Consuming enough protein also has been shown to enhance learning and intellectual development. Not only that, the zinc found in chicken, pork, and beef is beneficial to a healthy immune system. Likewise, the linoleic acid in meat may help prevent certain diseases, such as arthritis, breast cancer, and eczema.

However, since red meat is also a major source of saturated fat and cholesterol, choose wisely. What's best? It depends. Fat content varies with cut and grade. For example, white meat chicken is lower in fat than dark, and round and loin cuts of beef and pork are the most lean. Also, trimming off most visible fat before cooking significantly reduces the amount of saturated fat you eat, as does removing the skin on poultry. See the chart below for a comparison of fat content in different types of meat.

Meat and Poultry Fat Guide	
Meat/Poultry	**Grams of Fat (estimates based on 3½ oz.)**
Turkey, skinless, light meat, roasted	3.2
Chicken, skinless, light meat, roasted	4
Beef, top round, select cut, trimmed, broiled	5
Pork tenderloin, trimmed, roasted	5
Ham, fresh lean	5
Turkey, skinless, dark meat, roasted	7
Beef, tenderloin, select cut, trimmed, broiled	8
Chicken, skinless, dark meat, roasted	9
Hamburger, 80% lean	11
Goose/duck, skinless, roasted	12
Turkey bologna	16
Pork sausage	26
Hot dog	29
Beef bologna	29
Pork spare ribs	30

Fishing for Nutrients

Although often not a favorite with kids, fish is perhaps the most beneficial protein food. It contains the high-protein pluses of meat minus the saturated fat found in beef, pork, and poultry. Instead, it has important heart-healthy omega-3 fatty acids. Good omega-3 fats decrease risky triglycerides, inhibit damaging inflammation, help keep arteries clear, and improve blood vessel function. So try to work seafood—salmon, canned light tuna, oysters, herring, and cod—into your family's menu. According to recent research, even eating fish as seldom as three times per month can have a beneficial effect.

RealAge Projection: Children who develop a taste for fish and seafood are likely to make it a regular part of their adult diet. If they do, their RealAge could be 37 when they're turning 40.

Something's Fishy

The levels of mercury found in some fish is a growing concern, so limit or avoid shark, albacore tuna, and tuna steaks (canned light tuna is okay), swordfish, king mackerel, red snapper, and tilefish. Safer choices include salmon, sardines, pollock, and catfish.

If you're serving fish caught in local waters by family and friends—and if you're not sure about the level of mercury or other contaminants in your local lakes, rivers, and coastal areas—limit your family's consumption to about 6 ounces each per week.

For more information about the risks of mercury in seafood, visit the U.S. Food and Drug Administration's Center for Food Safety and Applied Nutrition at www.cfsan.fda.gov. Or call their toll-free line at 888-SAFEFOOD (888-723-3366).

What If Your Child Wants to Become a Vegetarian?

What would you do if your child suddenly decided to become a vegetarian or vegan? If you're a meat eater, you'd worry, right? About whether she'll get all the nutrients she needs if she cuts out foods you believe are essential? You might even attempt to forbid it, or dismiss it as a youthful whim.

For most kids, the decision to become a vegetarian or vegan is a thoughtful one, based on ethical concerns about animals and the planet, or health issues, or both. Even if it seems to be just a phase or an assertion of independence, this lifestyle choice deserves respect and support.

First, you need to determine how far she plans to go in excluding certain foods:

- Lacto-ovo vegetarians eat eggs and dairy products.
- Ovo vegetarians eat eggs but no dairy.
- Vegans don't eat foods that are derived from any animal source, so eggs and dairy are not included. Because vegan diets are so restrictive, it can be difficult to meet the nutritional and caloric needs of a growing child.

Educating yourself and your child about this way of eating is critical. You must provide alternatives for foods that have been eliminated, and be sure that your novice vegetarian is getting enough of the vital nutrients needed for overall health.

The major concern is protein. But by pairing certain foods, your child can get the total protein that is found in meat. For instance, combining either legumes (e.g., beans, lentils) with whole grains or seeds, or dairy products with grains, creates a complete protein. Eggs also contain complete protein, but don't rely on them exclusively.

If your child "goes vegan"—that is, eliminates all animal products, including milk, eggs, and cheese—encourage her to eat plenty of fresh, dark green veggies for iron, B vitamins, and other minerals, and to drink soy milk fortified with vitamin B_{12} and calcium. Soy- and other vegetable-based meat alternatives are now widely available, so stock your freezer with these healthy protein sources.

For a comprehensive look at vegetarian and vegan diets, read one of the many books on the topic.

How many times per month does your child participate in choosing healthy foods for dinner?

Good nutritional habits come from more than just eating. Kids should also be involved in the selection, preparation, and presentation of meals. It's the best way to teach them about healthy food. You can start as early as age 3 with activities such as adding dry ingredients to a mixing bowl and helping to choose foods at the grocery store.

Yes, it can be a hassle to take kids to the supermarket. They squirm in the cart or disappear down the aisle; they get bored, bicker, and ask for all kinds of tempting junk food. You'd probably rather leave them at home. But if you do, your kids won't learn how to shop smart, and that's a lesson they can't afford to miss. So try some of these shopping tips:

- **Be a taskmaster.** Give each child a job to do—finding items on the shopping list or wrapping the twist ties around the produce bags. Older kids can manage coupons. Keep them busy, and they'll have less time to pester each other, and you.
- **Celebrate something old, something new.** To help get a wide variety of healthy foods into the family diet, let each

child select an old favorite and then pick out something that they've never tried before.

- **Let teens be chef for a day.** Have them choose a recipe ahead of time and then put them in charge of collecting the ingredients and preparing the dish for the family to try.
- **Make a game of it.** Tell young children that the family is going to eat a rainbow, and have them choose fruits and vegetables from every color group.
- **Bring munchies.** Pack a snack to keep children happy, not hungry and cranky, while shopping.
- **Put them in control.** If your children are old enough to maneuver a kid-sized cart around the store, give them five items to find for their cart. Just be sure to teach them the rules of the road first!
- **Give 'em label lessons.** Teach your kids how to compare labels. For example, have them check a few different loaves to find the one with the most fiber. Showing children why certain foods are better than others will benefit their health for years to come.

Dr. Jen's Fresh Family Outings

"Each season, my family and I visit a farm that lets us pick our own apples, peaches, pumpkins, or berries. It's become a tradition, and we've started inviting friends to join us. We took it a step further last summer and planted a small vegetable garden of our own. Besides improving our meals, it's been a great way to spend fun time together as a family—and it's even great exercise."

Giving kids the power to make some decisions about food makes healthy eating easier and more enjoyable for everyone.

Oh, one more thing: A stunning 24,000 kids wound up in the ER in 2005 as a result of shopping-cart accidents. If possible, don't put your child in a front-basket seat. Instead, look for carts with molded low-down child seats attached to them (these often look like cars). They are far safer than regular wire carts. And never put infant carriers on top of a shopping cart. Instead, use one of those strap-on chest carriers that holds your baby against your body, leaving your arms free.

How about meal preparation—does your child help out?
Kids tend to get overexcited right before dinnertime. They've had some downtime from school, done their homework, and

Kids ages 3 and up can:

- **Fetch** ingredients from the refrigerator or cupboard
- **Tear** up lettuce for a salad
- **Snap** green beans and pea pods
- **Decorate** the table—paper placemats and crayons are all they need

Kids ages 6 and up can:

- **Peel** vegetables like cucumbers and potatoes
- **Shred** cheese
- **Grate** carrots
- **Mash** yams or potatoes for, as my kids say, smashed potatoes
- **Shuck** corn on the cob
- **Read** recipe instructions aloud to you (helps reading skills, too)
- **Assemble** sandwiches and salads
- **Measure** dry and wet ingredients (sneak in a little math while they're at it)

Kids ages 8 and up can:

- **Chop** vegetables
- **Plan** a meal
- **Follow** simple recipes
- **And finally,** do the dishes (start with unbreakable pans)

may be anxious for a parent to arrive home from work. This is a great time to focus their energy on helping with the meal.

Even toddlers can be given a job to do—something as simple as putting napkins on the table. Older kids can stir sauces or, with supervision, chop vegetables. Teenagers who like to cook can prepare a whole dish or even a whole meal once a week.

Make sure the task is age-appropriate (no sharp or pointed utensils for little ones). Thank them for their efforts and overlook the less-than-perfect. Who cares if a recipe doesn't turn out perfectly, or a little milk is spilled in the pouring? Keep the goal in mind: family fun and healthy habits.

Making meal preparation a family activity has multiple rewards. You'll find that putting kids in charge of a few things makes them more likely to enjoy mealtimes together. It also makes cooking less of a chore for you, so you're more likely to make a homemade meal rather than dialing out for pizza again (which is allowed sometimes, too!). Plus, kids are more likely to eat dishes—even unusual ones—they helped create.

How often do you sit down as a family and eat together?
Ideally, seven days a week, but I know that isn't realistic. What with gymnastics on Mondays, soccer on Tuesdays, swimming on Thursdays—and your own book-group meetings on Fridays—sitting down together for dinner isn't always possible.

Still, try to schedule a family dinner several times a week, and some family breakfasts, too. Even kids who resist usually wind up enjoying getting parents' undivided attention to talk about their day. Making family meals a daily habit that children look forward to helps them develop healthier attitudes about food (and also discourages destructive weight-loss behaviors).

Keep meals lively by ending with a joke or riddle to solve by the next meal. Have everyone share something that went well or not so well that day. This routine helps build strong family relationships that last a lifetime.

When ... does your family/child usually eat dinner?

Studi... ...amilies have
healt... ...ious foods—
if par... ...ating habits.
Key ...

-
-

...eat while watching TV— ...ational programs—tend to ...fruits and vegetables, more ...ls and sodas, and more cal- ...ably because they focus on ...e watching, not what they're ...nd familiar?

Wa...

Ok... ...our family is
sitti... ...d tasty meal
tha... ...pare. Should
you...

... notion that
des... ...ids to eat even
when they're full... ...can nurture an
overeater and lead to weight problems later in life.

Your child should learn to recognize what fullness feels like and know when to stop eating. If you're worried about wasting food, just serve children realistic portions. If it's not enough, they can always get a second helping. And make dessert an exception, not the rule, and not a reward for eating every bite.

Does your child take a multivitamin regularly?

A daily multi can ensure a child meets most minimum requirements for vitamins and minerals. However, a child who eats a balanced diet probably doesn't need a multi, especially since so many foods kids eat are now fortified with vitamins and minerals. Also, a pill is no substitute for nutritious food. At the same time, getting a balanced diet into kids week in, week out, can be challenging—especially with picky eaters.

What about iron supplements to prevent anemia? In general, they probably aren't necessary because most kids eat enough iron-fortified foods. Still, I screen for anemia once a year until age 4. After that, it's usually not necessary except for girls who are menstruating. I usually advise their taking a multivitamin with iron to supplement their iron intake.

Some kids are highly likely to need specific vitamin/mineral supplements:

- Premature babies
- Vegetarians/vegans
- Children who can't tolerate certain foods (e.g., dairy or wheat)
- Chronically ill children
- Adolescent girls
- Exclusively breast-fed babies
- Kids who live in very northern areas and get little sunlight during many months

Hint: Vitamin C helps the body absorb iron. So try to pair iron-rich veggies (beans, spinach) or iron-fortified grains (many breads and cereals) with foods that are high in vitamin C (citrus, berries, melons, tomatoes, yams, etc.). But avoid combining tea or milk with iron-rich foods; both hinder the mineral's absorption.

Small Changes, Big Rewards

I want to emphasize the fact that I don't expect you to make all the changes suggested in this chapter, or that you need to. It's impossible to be perfect when it comes to feeding kids. But I do hope you've come away with a better understanding of what good, balanced nutrition is, how diet can affect children in both the short- and long-term, and good ways to start them down the road of healthier eating.

Even making just one change—like getting a good breakfast into your kids each morning—will make a big difference, and one success may lead to others. Who knows? Perhaps you'll start packing a lunch for your child on most days, or preparing more dinners from wholesome ingredients and ordering less takeout. When you see how these changes improve your child's energy level, behavior, school performance, and, if it's an issue, weight—well, there's no better motivation.

Daily Nutritional Recommendations for Boys, 7 months–18 years

These recommendations are based on the Dietary Reference Intakes developed by the Institute of Medicine of the National Academies. The amounts listed indicate the levels that meet the minimum nutrient requirements of nearly all healthy children in each age group. **ND** indicates that no recommendation has been determined due to lack of data.

Use this as a guide for building a healthful daily diet for your child. If a range is listed, aim to stay within the two levels, offering a variety of foods that contain that nutrient.

MACRONUTRIENTS

Nutrient	7–12 mo	1–3 y	4–8 y	9–13 y	14–18 y	Sample Food Sources
Protein	13.5 g	13 g	19 g	34 g	52 g	tuna, canned or fresh; chicken breast; beef; turkey; salmon; garbanzo beans; milk; yogurt; tofu; cottage cheese; eggs
Carbohydrate	95 g	130 g	130 g	130 g	130 g	fruits; vegetables; beans and lentils; high-fiber whole grains (such as whole-wheat bread, oatmeal, brown rice, whole-wheat pasta, whole-grain cereals, and other products made with whole-grain flours rather than refined or "white" flour)
Total Fiber	ND	19 g	25 g	31 g	38 g	beans and lentils; whole-grain cereals; nuts; raspberries; whole-wheat bread (100%); sunflower seeds; apples; blueberries; green peas; pears; sweet potatoes w/skin, baked; white potatoes w/skin, baked; brown rice; broccoli; nectarines

HEALTHY FATS						
n-6 PUFA (omega-6s or linoleic acid)	4.6 g	7 g	10 g	12 g	16 g	eggs; poultry; whole-grain breads; plant-based margarine and oils (such as sunflower, corn, safflower, olive, canola)
n-3 PUFA (omega-3s or a-linolenic acid)	0.5 g	0.7 g	0.9 g	1.2 g	1.6 g	cold-water fish, including salmon, trout, tuna (fresh and canned), Atlantic mackerel, sardines, Pacific herring, and most shellfish
VITAMINS & MINERALS						
Nutrient	**7–12 mo**	**1–3 y**	**4–8 y**	**9–13 y**	**14–18 y**	**Sample Food Sources**
Vitamin A	500–600 mcg	300–600 mcg	400–900 mcg	600–1,700 mcg	900–2,800 mcg	carrots, raw; sweet potatoes; cantaloupe; pumpkin, canned; spinach; mangoes; swordfish; enriched bran or wheat flakes; winter squash
Vitamin C	50 mg	15–400 mg	25–650 mg	45–1,200 mg	75–1,800 mg	red and green bell peppers; papayas; strawberries; oranges; orange juice; tomatoes; tomato juice; cantaloupe; Brussels sprouts; mangoes; broccoli; honeydew melon; watermelon
Vitamin D	5–25 mcg	5–50 mcg	5–50 mcg	5–50 mcg	5–50 mcg	Atlantic mackerel; evaporated milk; milk, low-fat and fortified; Atlantic cod; granola; raisin bran; corn flakes; eggs

VITAMINS & MINERALS					
Vitamin E	5 mg	6–200 mg	7–300 mg	11–300 mg	15–300 mg	almonds; hazelnuts; sweet potatoes; safflower oil; peanut butter; avocados; mangoes; corn oil; asparagus; pears; apples
Vitamin K	2.5 mcg	30 mcg	55 mcg	60 mcg	75 mcg	kale; swiss chard; spinach; cabbage; broccoli; red leaf lettuce; olive oil
Vitamin B_6	0.3 mg	0.5–30 mg	0.6–40 mg	1.0–60 mg	1.3–80 mg	chicken, light meat; banana; tomato paste; sunflower seeds; turkey, light meat; ground beef; crab meat; artichokes; sweet potatoes; pork; tuna; sole; sardines; cod; haddock
Folate (B_9)	80 mcg	150–300 mcg	200–400 mcg	300–600 mcg	400–800 mcg	asparagus; artichokes; Brussels sprouts; black-eyed peas; sunflower seeds; apples; lima beans; soybeans; avocados; spinach; broccoli; bananas; oranges
Vitamin B_{12}	0.5 mcg	0.9 mcg	1.2 mcg	1.8 mcg	2.4 mcg	salmon; tuna; beef, roast or ground; lamb; enriched bran or wheat flakes; sole; haddock; pancakes from mix; cod; fish sticks; swordfish; yogurt; milk; macaroni and cheese; eggs
Calcium	270 mg	500–2,500 mg	800–2,500 mg	1,300–2,500 mg	1,300–2,500 mg	yogurt; cheese; macaroni and cheese; eggnog; fortified soymilk; milk; pink salmon, canned; kale; spinach; broccoli; tofu

VITAMINS & MINERALS						
Iron	11–40 mg	7–40 mg	10–40 mg	8–40 mg	11–45 mg	enriched bran flakes; enriched wheat farina; clams; enriched wheat flakes; wheat bran; whole-grain wheat flour; lentils; spinach
Magnesium	75 mg	80 mg	130 mg	240 mg	410 mg	tofu; soybeans; cashews; tomato paste; salmon; spinach; oatmeal; peanuts; baked potatoes, white or sweet; fortified cereals (bran or wheat); shrimp; brown rice; watermelon
Phosphorus	275 mg	460–3,000 mg	500–3,000 mg	1,250–4,000 mg	1,250–4,000 mg	bran flakes; pancakes; chili with beans; pinto beans; milk; rib-eye beef steak; almonds; oatmeal; eggs
Potassium	700 mg	3,000 mg	3,800 mg	4,500 mg	4,700 mg	tomato paste; dried peaches; baked potatoes; sole; salmon; sardines; cod; watermelon; cantaloupe; honeydew; dried apricots; scallops; bananas; grapefruit juice; yogurt; chestnuts; milk; artichokes
Selenium	20–60 mcg	20–90 mcg	30–150 mcg	40–280 mcg	55–400 mcg	enriched bran flakes; turkey; ham; beef; lamb; pork
Zinc	3–5 mg	3–7 mg	5–12 mg	8–23 mg	11–34 mg	turkey, dark meat; enriched bran flakes; ham; beef; lamb; pork; lobster; black-eyed peas; shrimp; chicken, light meat; yogurt
mcg = micrograms; mg = milligrams; g = grams						

Daily Nutritional Recommendations for Girls, 7 months–18 years

These recommendations are based on the Dietary Reference Intakes developed by the Institute of Medicine of the National Academies. The amounts listed indicate the levels that meet the minimum nutrient requirements of nearly all healthy children in each age group. **ND** indicates that no recommendation has been determined due to lack of data.

Use this as a guide for building a healthful daily diet for your child. If a range is listed, aim to stay within the two levels, offering a variety of foods that contain that nutrient.

MACRONUTRIENTS						
Nutrient	**7–12 mo**	**1–3 y**	**4–8 y**	**9–13 y**	**14–18 y**	**Sample Food Sources**
Protein	13.5 g	13 g	19 g	34 g	46g	tuna, canned or fresh; chicken breast; beef; turkey; salmon; garbanzo beans; milk; yogurt; tofu; cottage cheese; eggs
Carbohydrate	95 g	130 g	130 g	130 g	130 g	fruits; vegetables; beans and lentils; high-fiber whole grains (such as whole-wheat bread, oatmeal, brown rice, whole-wheat pasta, whole-grain cereals, and other products made with whole-grain flours rather than refined or "white" flour)
Total Fiber	ND	19 g	25 g	26 g	26 g	beans and lentils; whole-grain cereals; nuts; raspberries; whole-wheat bread (100%); sunflower seeds; apples; blueberries; green peas; pears; sweet potatoes w/skin, baked; white potatoes w/skin, baked; brown rice; broccoli; nectarines

HEALTHY FATS						
n-6 PUFA (omega-6s or linoleic acid)	4.6 g	7 g	10 g	10 g	11 g	eggs; poultry; whole-grain breads; plant-based margarine and oils (such as sunflower, corn, safflower, olive, canola)
n-3 PUFA (omega-3s or a-linolenic acid)	0.5 g	0.7 g	0.9 g	1.0 g	1.1 g	cold-water fish, including salmon, trout, tuna (fresh and canned), Atlantic mackerel, sardines, Pacific herring, and most shellfish
VITAMINS AND MINERALS						
Nutrient	**7–12 mo**	**1–3 y**	**4–8 y**	**9–13 y**	**14–18 y**	**Sample Food Sources**
Vitamin A	500–600 mcg	300–600 mcg	400–900 mcg	600–1,700 mcg	700–2,800 mcg	carrots, raw; sweet potatoes; cantaloupe; pumpkin, canned; spinach; mangoes; swordfish; enriched bran or wheat flakes; winter squash
Vitamin C	50 mg	15–400 mg	25–650 mg	45–1,200 mg	65–1,800 mg	red and green bell peppers; papaya; strawberries; oranges; orange juice; tomatoes; tomato juice; cantaloupe; Brussels sprouts; mangoes; broccoli; honeydew melon; watermelon
Vitamin D	5–25 mcg	5–50 mcg	5–50 mcg	5–50 mcg	5–50 mcg	Atlantic mackerel; evaporated milk; milk, low-fat and fortified; Atlantic cod; granola; raisin bran; corn flakes; eggs
Vitamin E	5 mg	6–200 mg	7–300 mg	11–300 mg	15–300 mg	almonds; hazelnuts; sweet potatoes; safflower oil; peanut butter; avocados; mangoes; corn oil; asparagus; pears; apples

VITAMINS AND MINERALS						
Vitamin K	2.5 mcg	30 mcg	55 mcg	60 mcg	75 mcg	kale; swiss chard; spinach; cabbage; broccoli; red leaf lettuce; olive oil
Vitamin B$_6$	0.3 mg	0.5–30 mg	0.6–40 mg	1.0–60 mg	1.3–80 mg	chicken, light meat; banana; tomato paste; sunflower seeds; turkey, light meat; ground beef; crab meat; artichokes; sweet potatoes; pork; tuna; sole; sardines; cod; haddock
Folate (B$_9$)	80 mcg	150–300 mcg	200–400 mcg	300–600 mcg	400–800 mcg	asparagus; artichokes; Brussels sprouts; black-eyed peas; sunflower seeds; apples; lima beans; soybeans; avocados; spinach; broccoli; bananas; oranges
Vitamin B$_{12}$	0.5 mcg	0.9 mcg	1.2 mcg	1.8 mcg	2.4 mcg	salmon; tuna; beef, roast or ground; lamb; enriched bran or wheat flakes; sole; haddock; pancakes from mix; cod; fish sticks; swordfish; yogurt; milk; macaroni and cheese; eggs
Calcium	270 mg	500–2,500 mg	800–2,500 mg	1,300–2,500 mg	1,300–2,500 mg	yogurt; cheese; macaroni and cheese; eggnog; fortified soymilk; milk; pink salmon, canned; kale; spinach; broccoli; tofu
Iron	11–40 mg	7–40 mg	10–40 mg	8–40 mg	15–45 mg	enriched bran flakes; enriched wheat farina; clams; enriched wheat flakes; wheat bran; whole-grain wheat flour; lentils; spinach

VITAMINS AND MINERALS						
Magnesium	75 mg	80 mg	130 mg	240 mg	360 mg	tofu; soybeans; cashews; tomato paste; salmon; spinach; oatmeal; peanuts; baked potatoes, white or sweet; fortified cereals (bran or wheat); shrimp; brown rice; watermelon
Phosphorus	275 mg	460–3,000 mg	500–3,000 mg	1,250–4,000 mg	1,250–4,000 mg	bran flakes; pancakes; chili with beans; pinto beans; milk; rib-eye beef steak; almonds; oatmeal; eggs
Potassium	700 mg	3,000 mg	3,800 mg	4,500 mg	4,700 mg	tomato paste; dried peaches; baked potatoes; sole; salmon; sardines; cod; watermelon; cantaloupe; honeydew; dried apricots; scallops; bananas; grapefruit juice; yogurt; chestnuts; milk; artichokes
Selenium	20–60 mcg	20–90 mcg	30–150 mcg	40–280 mcg	55–400 mcg	enriched bran flakes; turkey; ham; beef; lamb; pork
Zinc	3–5 mg	3–7 mg	5–12 mg	8–23 mg	9–34 mg	turkey, dark meat; enriched bran flakes; ham; beef; lamb; pork; lobster; black-eyed peas; shrimp; chicken, light meat; yogurt
mcg = micrograms; mg = milligrams; g = grams						

Many of the charts and checklists in this chapter can be printed out at
www.RealAge.com/parenting

Chapter 3

SHAPE UP
Getting Kids to Play More than Video Games
(even that 9-year-old Nintendo nut)

TV. Cell phones. Video games. E-mails. Instant messages. iPods. With all of the electronics now available to children, a kid could live on the couch and never be bored. What's even more alarming is that so many other things discourage physical activity:

- School phys ed (PE) programs have been squeezed out by budget cuts or added curriculum requirements: Only *one* state requires daily PE.
- Instead of walking or biking to and from school, kids get driven for distance or safety reasons.
- There are fewer places to safely ride bikes, roller-skate, and skateboard.
- There are fewer places to play impromptu games of hide-and-seek, Frisbee, or softball.

IMMEDIATE BENEFITS OF EXERCISE	LONG-TERM BENEFITS OF EXERCISE
• Better sleep	• Stronger bones, joints, and muscles
• Better mood	• Reduced feelings of anxiety
• More energy, less fatigue	• Less risk of depression
• Fewer aches and pains	• Better sense of well-being
• Fewer colds	• Less stress
• More strength, stamina, and flexibility	• Healthier body weight
• Better focus and attention span	• Reduced risk of heart disease, colon cancer, and type 2 diabetes
	• Lower cholesterol
	• Lower blood pressure

But your child's world doesn't have to be limited. Moms, dads, think back to being a kid. Think about those times when you would get totally absorbed in building forts. Chasing lightning bugs. Playing tag. Riding bikes. Rediscover that playful spirit and share it with your kids.

> Almost 50 percent of 12- to 21-year-olds are not active enough.

Join in, or even get things started. You know how contagious it is to watch someone who's having a blast? Your children will notice and want to be part of it.

The Payoff Is Huge

Kids who lead an active physical life get all the short- and long-term benefits listed above, plus they have fewer behavioral problems, form stronger friendships, and are just happier and better adjusted.

Group activities also encourage self-discipline, sportsmanship, leadership, and the ability to get along with others—skills that will serve kids well all their life. In addition, staying fit helps children feel good about themselves and builds self-confidence.

Fight the Competition

So, how do you pry your child away from that latest version of Tomb Raider, EverQuest, or Super Mario? How do you convince a youngster to stop chatting online and go outside to play? How do you respond to a child who begs for just one more episode of *SpongeBob SquarePants*? (And why would you even consider saying no if they are quiet and occupied? I know you don't want to admit it, but believe me, you're not the only guilty parent.)

> Thirty-four percent of kids ages 12 to 19 would flunk an eight-minute treadmill test.

The answer is by doing, not saying. Be a role model. If you thrive on the benefits of physical activity, you're likely to pass on that positive attitude to your child.

This chapter will show you exactly how to break through the barriers and get kids exercising without their realizing that they're exercising. You'll definitely need to use your imagination to keep kids active through all the growing-up years. And remember, being a great role model is the most powerful tool you have! Let the 4 Is help you and your child get started.

> **The Research Proves It:**
> **Exercise Is the Key to a Long Life**
>
> To test the effect of exercise on kids who carry excess pounds, a group of overweight children ages 9 to 12 were put on a diet for a year—but some also started an exercise program.
>
> After only six weeks, pretty much all of them had lower cholesterol levels and healthier waist–hip ratios. The exercisers, however, also had less body fat and multiple improvements in their cardiovascular system.
>
> Translation? The exercisers will probably live longer.

1. **Identify: Get a handle on the situation**

   Identify and overcome barriers to physical activity . . . from disabilities and time constraints to excuses and safety issues.

2. **Inform: Find out what's out there**

   Explore exercise options at school—during PE, recess, club activities, team sports, individual sports, or activity time.

3. **Instruct: Be a "coach"**

   Work with your kids to help them learn new skills, and have fun doing it. But don't go overboard. There's a healthy balance between too little and too much exercise.

4. **Instill: Stick with it**

   Keep it up—parents and kids alike: Ditch the excuses and avoid the activity thieves like the TV and telephone. Put fitness first; there's always time for the other stuff.

Still feel daunted? Use the tips throughout this chapter; they've worked for me and my kids and patients.

What is the total time per day your child spends watching TV, movies, or playing video games?

Were you surprised when you added up the actual amount of time your child spends in front of a screen? You're not alone.

Nearly 50 percent of 8- to 16-year-olds watch three to five hours of TV each day. In a twelve-hour day, if six hours are spent at school and three to five are in front of a screen, that doesn't leave much time for shooting hoops or in-line skating. Kids' bodies are healthier

> Fifty percent of 8- to 16-year-olds spend three to five hours daily watching TV.

when they move on a regular basis; don't let them spend this many hours sitting still.

The Long-Term Picture of Screen Time

Kids who flop on the couch or in front of a computer game every chance they get are heading for a sedentary life. And I'm going to say this a million times because it's so true: A sedentary life will jeopardize your child's health, now and later.

Too much TV during childhood has been linked to adult obesity, a bad body image, and high cholesterol. And it's not just the lack of activity. It's what's on the screen. An average child sees 20,000 commercials each year, and the most common are for sugar-laden cereals, candy, sodas, and fat-packed snack foods. Today, children know all about Cocoa Puffs before they ever hear of asparagus.

> The average child watches 20,000 commercials each year, inevitably influencing values and desires.

As for time on the computer, sure, good computer skills are essential for today's kids. However, try to keep computer time that's not school-related to a maximum of an hour a day and schedule equal time for physical activity. To help regulate TV and computer time, try this approach:

- **Plan ahead:** Together, choose programs your child can watch, then turn the TV off before the next show begins. Similarly, pick out one DVD; when it's over, turn off the player. Choose one video game and agree on time limits before the game begins.
- **Watch together:** Help your child understand and process what he/she sees and hears on TV, games, and the Internet—from ads to lyrics (expect to have your eyes opened, too).

- **Hide the remote:** It's much harder to mindlessly flip through channels without one.
- **Minimize the sets:** Allow only one or two TVs in the house, and never put one in a child's bedroom or in eating areas!

True Parenting Story: A Summertime Battle Over TV

Summer vacation had just begun. After a long and busy school year, I was excited to have my daughters, Nikki and Wendy, at home with me. I had fun plans: the zoo, story time at the public library, picnics, lots of playground time, the new children's museum—and I even scheduled a couple of art classes for them.

Well, that first Monday morning, my girls woke up and headed straight for the TV. They had the morning's show schedule all planned out. *SpongeBob SquarePants* at 7:00 a.m., an hour of *Jimmy Neutron,* then a couple of Disney shows and Cartoon Network. I shrugged my shoulders and let it slide. It was their first day off, after all. But the following morning, it was the same thing all over again. I asked the girls to turn off the TV and get dressed so we could go to the park, but they moaned, "Just one show, please?" We finally left, but not without a battle.

I'd had enough. Late that night, I unplugged the TV. In the morning, after Wendy unsuccessfully attempted to turn it on, she called out, "Mom! I think the TV is broken!"

"It is?" I innocently replied. "Oh, too bad. Well, how about we go to the zoo?" Our TV remained "broken" all summer long.

—KAREN, OLD TAPPAN, NJ

Okay, Karen wasn't totally honest with her children, and maybe you'd take a different approach, but the point is not to get side-railed by TV demands. Karen later told me how Nikki

> ### Five Steps to a More Active Lifestyle
>
> Here are some ways to move your child happily from the TV and computer and toward more active hobbies.
>
> **1. Get classy.** Enroll your child in a dance class, or karate, or diving lessons.
>
> **2. Tour the town.** Explore different neighborhoods together.
>
> **3. Join the team. Or don't.** Encourage your child to try out for soccer, softball, swimming or—if team sports don't suit—to try individual activities such as biking and skating.
>
> **4. Hit the trail.** Research opportunities for hiking in your area.
>
> **5. Take a learning adventure.** Plan trips to museums, galleries, and historical sites.

and Wendy raced each other at the zoo to see the polar bears . . . so I think this little white lie was worth it.

How does your child spend downtime?

You were asked to choose two answers that best applied to your child. Use the chart to compare yours to other families.

Unless at least one of your answers was "playing actively," help your child get more unstructured activity. "Unstructured" means no strict rules, no umpires, no tutors, no coaches. Let kids create games that work for them. Scavenger hunts, obstacle courses, and three-legged races are all high-energy fun. Sure, adults may need to supervise, but they shouldn't interfere just because "official" rules are not being followed . . . especially if everyone is having fun.

Sometimes unplanned activities are the most natural. Your child may love to come home from school and throw sticks for the dog, play stickball, ride scooters, or climb trees. After sitting in class all day, it doesn't matter what a kid does, as long as it's active.

How RealAge Kids Spend Their Downtime

Healthy Kids Test	Other Parents of Kids Aged:						
Answers	**0–2**	**3–4**	**5–7**	**8–10**	**11–13**	**14–16**	**17+**
Watching TV (shows, movies, DVDs)	38%	63%	54%	53%	54%	52%	49%
Playing video games	0%	4%	16%	29%	33%	28%	22%
Using the computer (surfing the Web, playing games, chatting online)	0%	7%	9%	12%	25%	42%	42%
Reading (books, magazines)	14%	11%	12%	20%	21%	19%	18%
Crafts (drawing, painting, models)	2%	10%	13%	8%	5%	3%	4%
Playing in his/her room	35%	36%	33%	21%	11%	5%	3%
Playing actively outdoors	28%	32%	40%	42%	36%	24%	19%
Playing actively indoors	60%	34%	20%	11%	8%	7%	9%
Other	8%	3%	2%	2%	4%	10%	12%
Statistics gathered from RealAge Healthy Kids Test online, www.RealAge.com/parenting.							

Give the Gift of Fitness

Use birthdays and holidays as a way to encourage kids to get moving. Fitness-minded gifts are also a great way to introduce an active hobby; for instance, you could outfit a teenager for rock climbing. A home version of Dance Dance Revolution (DDR) will get your video-game player stepping to the music. Try a fitness-center membership or a trial lesson in a new activity. Check out sports camps or clinics in summer or on school vacation.

Downtime Ideas

Water play
Squirt toys
Water balloons
Slip 'N Slide

Playground fun
Jump rope
Hopscotch
Two-square
Jungle gym

Lawn games
Horseshoes
Badminton
Frisbee

Backyard favorites
Hide-and-seek
Tag
Simon Says
Red Light, Green Light
Keep-away

Overcoming Obstacles to Activity

At this point you're probably thinking, "I know my child should be more active, but . . ." It's true that some kids prefer quiet, seated activities to more rambunctious ones. When playing outside, they may sit down on the grass and study a ladybug while the others race around the yard. That's fine. At least they're outdoors and actively engaged in something, not staring at a flickering screen.

But there are other real barriers to an active lifestyle that I see in my practice every day. They include:

- **Lack of energy,** which can be triggered by poor sleep, poor nutrition, or a medical problem. If your child seems chronically low on energy, a checkup may be in order.
- **Lack of motivation,** which can be caused by poor role-modeling on your part, peer pressure, limited options, or burnout. If you suspect that a lack of motivation is your doing, it's definitely time to reevaluate your lifestyle. Make more family activity a priority. You'll be helping your kids—and yourself.
- **Time constraints,** due to an overcrowded or erratic schedule.
- **Social factors,** such as shyness, low self-esteem, or lack of confidence in athletic abilities. (See Chapter 6 for help here.)
- **Environmental barriers,** such as extreme weather conditions, limited parks or yards, and unsafe neighborhoods. Encourage indoor play by:

- "Sock skating" on bare floors (or do the real thing at an indoor rink)
- Stocking an open room with foam balls and baskets, Twister, dance videos, and Chinese jump rope
- Play-wrestling in a pile of pillows and cushions
- Listening to up-tempo music and dancing
- Putting on a play, puppet show, or concert
- Seeking out community centers, indoor gyms, or shopping centers that have climbing walls, balls, hoops, and other kid-friendly equipment

Once you have figured out the barriers, you can start focusing on ways to overcome them. Remember that every kid is wired differently and has certain physical characteristics that make him/her better at some things than others. The key is to tap into those strengths and find activities that allow your child to shine.

If your child is artsy, try a nature walk to collect pinecones and leaves for a collage. Take an animal lover bird watching. A bookworm can walk, bike, or skate to the local library. Kids who are more "mathlete" than athlete can use their math skills to create superfast paper airplanes and then head to the park for a fly-off. New computer-based games that marry technology and fitness are great for video-gamers. Instead of exercising only thumbs or fingers, these games get kids' hearts pounding. Some "exertainment" or "exergaming" machines simulate ski, car, or motorcycle races where the faster you pedal, the faster your racer goes on the screen. Others simulate boxing, Spider-Man moves, guitar playing, bongo drumming, and even karate!

How Much Physical Activity Should Your Child Get?

The chart on the following page shows the ideal amounts of exercise for a healthy child. If your child isn't active at all, build up to the recommended amount over three to six months. Start small, slow, and fun. If your child has any physical problems, check with your pediatrician for the optimal amounts.

RealAge Projection: Kids who learn to love being active when they're young are likely to stick with this healthy habit when they're adults. And if they do—getting a good mix of aerobic, strength, and flexibility exercise—at 35, their RealAge will really be more like 27.

At School: How to Count Up the Active Minutes

When people ask about your child's favorite subject in school, is the answer "Recess!"? That's not a bad answer, especially if your kid is sweaty and thirsty afterward. Recess is just as important as math and reading.

But have you dropped by school and watched recess from the other side of the fence? What if your child doesn't run around actively, or reads on a bench, or just walks along the sidelines, kicking pebbles? What if the school doesn't have recess, or if your child is in middle or high school and there's no phys ed? If that's the case, he or she probably isn't getting enough exercise. Ideally, kids should get half of their daily activity at school. If they don't, and aren't involved in sports, parents need to get them moving after school and on weekends.

If you're not sure about your child's activities at school, ask. Ask the teachers, too. Be sure that school-related activities:

- Focus more on fun than on competition
- Are designed to develop balance and coordination (dribbling, sprinting, and jumping rope all do this)
- Offer a mix of activities that appeal to different children

Daily Physical Activity Recommendations for Children, 7 months–18 years

Moderate exercise is any exercise that gets children moving, causing them to feel some exertion, but allowing them to carry on a conversation comfortably during the activity.

Vigorous exercise is any activity that is intense enough to be a challenge and results in a significant increase in heart and breathing rate.

Note: Depending on level of exertion and duration, some activities may be either moderate or vigorous, such as bicycling, dancing, etc.

Use this as a guide to help keep kids moving and active daily, or on most days of the week.

Age	Amount of Activity	Maximum Amount of Time Kids Should Spend Idle	Examples
7 months–1 year	At least 30 to 60 minutes of structured play centered around exploring the child's environment	NA	Playing peek-a-boo; performing finger and hand puppet shows; stacking blocks; crawling or toddling through an indoor obstacle course; playing drums with wooden spoons; rolling a soft ball back and forth; blowing bubbles; acting out nursery rhymes
2–4 years	60 minutes of moderate activity that builds balance and movement, and increases awareness of body space AND 30 to 60 minutes of vigorous activity	1 hour at a time of inactivity (except when sleeping)	Practicing basic tumbling moves; imitating animal movements (pouncing, jumping, creeping, crawling); playing hopscotch; tossing and kicking a beach ball; chasing bubbles; acting out plays or stories; singing songs and dancing along

Age	Amount of Activity	Maximum Amount of Time Kids Should Spend Idle	Examples
5–11 years	At least 60 minutes of moderate activity broken up by brief periods of rest AND Three or four 15-minute bouts of vigorous, age-appropriate activity	2 hours at a time of inactivity (except when sleeping)	Walking; dancing; bicycling; playground games; ice-skating or roller-skating; mowing the lawn; canoe-ing or kayaking; yoga; golfing; jogging or running; mountain biking; aerobic dance; martial arts; stair climbing; jumping rope; swimming; playing soccer; field hockey or ice hockey; lacrosse; tennis; volleyball; badminton; basketball; softball; baseball
12–20 years	30 to 60 minutes of moderate, age-appropriate activity AND 20 minutes of continuous activity that is moderate to vigorous		
These recommendations are based on guidelines developed by the National Association for Sport & Physical Education and the 1993 International Consensus Conference on Physical Activity.			

You can also download this chart at www.RealAge.com/parenting.

If the choice of school activities is slim, get involved. Join forces with other parents and school officials and give the phys ed program a healthy overhaul. Sometimes all it takes is a handful of suggestions to make a world of difference.

What is your child's most frequent mode of transportation?
Your answer may reveal a way to fit more exercise into your child's life:

- Is it safe for your child to walk or ride a skateboard to and from school instead of being driven?
- If not, could you and other parents participate in a "walking schoolbus," taking turns escorting a group of children to and from school? (Everyone benefits, kids *and* parents.)
- Could your grade-schooler ride a bike to a friend's house rather than being driven?
- Does your teen drive to practice when it's possible to walk or jog (and warm up in the process)?

Hoofing it can get kids into the habit of enjoying walking throughout life, even when a car is available. And when you absolutely have to drive them somewhere, park down the street from your destination and walk there together—it will give everyone a bit of fresh air and exercise before you arrive.

Which clubs, activities, or organizations does your child participate in regularly?
If you answered, "don't know," go find out! It's important to know what's important to your kid. Whether it's scouts, dance,

baseball, or volunteering as a junior lifeguard, these activities get your child up and moving. Even if the activity isn't active by itself, it might include some physical effort—a science club that occasionally goes rock collecting or caving, or a drama group that builds props and scenery.

Just be careful not to overschedule kids. A different activity each day of the week may result in children—and parents—who are overtired, overworked, and unmotivated. Kids need time to do homework, play, read, and rest. Allowing time for these will not only avoid activity burnout, but it'll save you from driving all over town, juggling a schedule that's even busier than yours. I try to limit my children to one or two activities at a time—swimming lessons and baseball in summer, for example, or snowboarding and hockey in the winter.

Use your judgment to determine whether your child is overscheduled. I find that when parents ask me if their kids' schedules are too full, they already know the answer is yes.

Team Spirit

Team sports are a classic way to get kids moving and may motivate them better than more solitary activities. Although winning shouldn't be the primary goal, being a part of a team can spur kids to work harder. If they work hard, they'll be in better shape; if they're in shape, their performance improves; if their performance improves, team performance improves. It's a healthy cycle, and one that should be encouraged. Team sports can help:

- Make exercise fun
- Build friendships
- Strengthen bones

- Improve cardiovascular health
- Build self-esteem
- Highlight teamwork
- Teach self-discipline and goal setting

Sports and Vitamins

Parents sometimes ask me to recommend a vitamin regimen for children who are involved with sports, hoping it will help athletic performance.

Take Andrew, for instance. At 14, he was growing fast. His caloric needs were up, as were his requirements for protein and vitamins A, C, E, B_6, folate, plus magnesium. Because he played basketball at school, his dad decided he should take multiple vitamin supplements. Besides giving him extra nutrients, maybe it would help his game as well.

Andrew's father and I had a discussion about vitamins—and other supplements that Andrew was interested in trying to enhance his ability on the court. I asked his dad to keep track of what Andrew was eating for a couple of days; after that, we'd talk more.

A few days later, his father called. Andrew's breakfast consisted of a large bowl of cereal, and after school, before practice, he ate an energy bar. Both items were fortified with vitamins and minerals in amounts greater than the RDA.

Caution! Overheating and Dehydration Are High Risks If Your Child Is:

- Playing in a very warm environment
- Out of shape or sedentary
- Overweight
- Recovering from an illness
- A consumer of large quantities of caffeinated beverages
- Someone who spends lots of time in air-conditioned rooms

Heat stroke is dangerous. If your child passes out, vomits, can't take in fluids, has chest or abdominal pain, or a temperature above 104, call 911.

Between those and the extra supplements he was taking, Andrew was exceeding his recommended daily requirements for iron, and vitamins A, C, E, and B$_6$. This wasn't good, since certain nutrients—including iron and fat-soluble vitamins like A, D, E, and K—can be toxic in excess amounts. Beyond the daily requirements needed to avoid illness and disease, any potential benefits to children are debatable.

> *RealAge Projection:* Tweens and teens who get into the habit of loading up on vitamins and supplements are likely to continue this habit as adults. If they do, rather than making them healthier, it could make their biological age almost 2 years older.

I suggested that Andrew take just a basic multi, continue eating fortified cereal for breakfast, and replace the energy bar with something less fortified but still healthy. A whole-wheat bagel or a snack bag of trail mix would be a good choice.

The Bottom Line

There is nothing wrong with wanting to excel at a chosen sport, but not everyone can be a star player. There is no scientific evidence that high doses of vitamins enhance athletic performance in children. In fact, they can be harmful. Beyond that worry, taking megadoses of anything suggests that pills can replace training and natural ability. As a parent, part of your job is to help your kids reach their full potential. The best way to do that is to encourage healthy eating and hard work.

Make sure your child really wants to play organized sports. For kids under 6, consider a team activity where everyone wins in the end and no score is kept. Most kids over 6 have a grasp of teamwork and may be interested in more competitive games. But children grow, mature, and learn skills at different rates and sometimes the physical and psychological demands of a team are too much for a child. Up until about age 11, kids are still figuring out how to build friendships. Although team sports do teach cooperation, winning and losing are also part of the game, and trying to beat friends on an opposing team can be confusing for some youngsters.

Battling the Burnout Barrier

A young athlete who gets tired and frustrated can get turned off from sports. The sport schedule may be overly rigorous, and initial enthusiasm may wane. To prevent burnout:

- Keep your focus (and your child's) on having fun and being part of a team, not on winning.
- Be careful to avoid using your young athlete's success to boost your own self-worth.
- Support and encourage, but don't pressure your child to perform.

How do you know if kids are ready for team competition? Ask yourself these questions:

- Do they show an interest?
- Is their emotional maturity similar to their teammates'? (How well do they accept defeat? How well do they take direction?)
- Are they big enough and coordinated enough to minimize injury?

Stay Hydrated During Hard Play

Kids should drink:

- 8 ounces (1 cup) of water approximately 30 minutes before activity begins
- 16–32 ounces (2–4 cups) of water for every hour of vigorous activity

If you're concerned, schedule a physical with a pediatrician before launching into sports season. You may find that it's better to delay, or that another activity is a better choice. Also, keep an eye out for warning signs that the experience is backfiring, such as a kid who constantly:

- Runs late for, or even skips, games and practices
- Complains of headaches or stomachaches before games

Also see the checklist at the end of this chapter for what coach(es) should know about your child.

Coaches Can Keep It Fun

Nearly half the kids who begin a sport eventually quit. They drop out for various reasons—injuries, too little game time, too much competition, or just not having fun. A good coach will recognize when children have too much pressure on them and balance competition with fun.

True Parenting Story: Beyond Organized Sports

From the moment Jackson was born, I looked forward to being a Little League dad. I planned to cheer from the bleachers, maybe even help coach.

Jackson enjoyed playing outside with his friends, but when the time came to sign up for T-ball, he showed no interest. I talked about other team sports and he just didn't seem enthused. I have to say I was disappointed, and a little worried about his fitness.

Now Jackson is 15 and a healthy outdoor-type guy. He loves to bike off-road with his friends. He spends hours each week skating around the neighborhood. Lately, he's been talking about learning to surf.

I used to worry that my son would miss out on something if he didn't join a team. I've realized that what's important is that he stays active and does what *he* enjoys doing.

—ROB, LONG ISLAND, NY

A Family Who Plays Together . . . Stays Active

Which family activities do you and your child enjoy on a frequent basis?

With the exception of reading books and watching movies, all the answers in the RealAge Healthy Kids Test offer great ways to stay active as a family. The trick is to tailor activities to your family, though if you have more than one child, occasionally plan one-on-one time with each of them. Some suggestions:

- **Take walks with a purpose.** This may seem so obvious that you've overlooked it. Identify trees, rocks, and plants. Make up a game, like finding all the blue houses, counting lampposts, or looking for a certain kind of flower. Tell stories as you walk. Or simply catch up on your child's life. Walking together allows the two of you to have heart-to-heart talks that might not happen otherwise.
- **Take your child along when you exercise.** If you go to a gym, ask if there are classes for kids. If you jog or bike, encourage older children to join you. Sign up for a bowling league, or train together for an everyone-wins "fun run."
- **Visit local parks.** Free fun, fresh air, and age-appropriate for everyone! Try to find and explore every park, playground, trail, and green space within a twenty-mile radius of your home.
- **Fly a kite.** Let your child pick out a kite, then fly it together. Or if you're feeling ambitious, build a kite together from scratch.
- **Plan an active vacation.** Take the family for a week—or even a day—to destinations that incorporate physical activity, such as kayaking, camping, exploring, sledding, and skating.

Take the Bore out of Chores

Ask your kids to rake leaves and the response will be underwhelming. Suggest jumping in a pile of leaves, and they'll probably beat you out the door. It's all in the presentation. Use your ingenuity to enlist help without their suspecting that it's anything but fun. Adding an element of competition—"Let's see who can pull the most weeds!"—also works well with many kids.

Of course this "two birds with one stone" approach often doesn't work with older kids. In those cases, don't belabor the benefits. That's about as effective as telling them that spinach will give them muscles like Popeye. Just insist that they complete assigned chores and smile to yourself, knowing that they're getting some exercise, too.

Use these ideas to help make chore time more like play time:

> **Plant a garden.** Involve children in preparing the soil and choosing and planting flowers, vegetables, and fruit. Have them help with weeding, watering, and harvesting. Then, take the kids to deliver baskets of food or flowers to neighbors.
>
> **Shovel snow.** Let children help with this winter chore. And play along the way—make snow angels or a fort or start a snowball fight. Afterward, go sledding for a reward (and more exercise).
>
> **Paint the fence.** Don't hesitate to let children help, but water-based paint is a good idea. Have younger kids paint pieces of wood on a drop cloth set out alongside the real project. A bucket of water will do as "paint" for the very young.
>
> **Care for a pet.** Take your kids and your dog to a park or beach where everyone can run around. Taking some

responsibility for a pet, from grooming to playing ball, will also help keep your child moving.

RealAge Projection: **A child who grows up with a family dog—and helps take care of it—will often become a dog owner as an adult. An adult who walks and plays with a dog on most days can make her RealAge at least one year younger.**

Start Today

Your child doesn't have to try playing ice hockey equipped like a pro or sign up for a year's worth of dance lessons. In fact, consider the time and money involved before jumping in with both feet. Try to set up one or two trial classes. That way, if it turns out that the activity isn't right, it's no big deal to switch. The point is just to get started, because an active lifestyle is the number one way to ensure a long, healthy life.

What the Coach Needs to Know About Your Kid

When kids begin a new sports program, there are some vital things the coach/instructor should know about them. This crib sheet makes it easy.

☐ Name _____

☐ Birth date _____

☐ Results of your child's sports physical, to determine overall health and readiness

_____

☐ Expectations—is this strictly for enjoyment or part of a long-term plan to achieve a high level of competence?

_____

☐ Any health limitations, such as asthma or epilepsy _____

☐ Any injuries that might impede performance _____

☐ Any allergies _____

☐ Child's doctors' names and contact information

   ☐ Name _____ Phone number _____

   ☐ Name _____ Phone number _____

Emergency contact information for parents and another responsible adult, in case parents can't be reached

   ☐ Name _____ Phone number _____

      ☐ Relationship to child _____

   ☐ Name _____ Phone number _____

      ☐ Relationship to child _____

   ☐ Name _____ Phone number _____

      ☐ Relationship to child _____

☐ Insurance provider and policy number _____

_____

☐ Any commitments your child has that might interfere with practices or games

_____

☐ Any additional information _____

_____

Things to Consider When Evaluating Your Child's Coach(es)

Background	• How extensive is the coach's experience within the sport? • Has the coach undergone a thorough background check? • Is the coach a good role model? Does he/she motivate and inspire the team?
Coaching style	• How competitive or laid back is the coach? Will that approach mesh or clash with your child's attitude? • Does the coach vigilantly follow rules, regulations, and proper techniques? • What is the practice schedule like? Will it fit your child's schedule?
Safety concerns	• Is the coach certified in CPR? • Does the coach lead warm-up exercises before practices and games to lessen the possibility of injury? • Does the coach encourage extreme diets or performance-enhancing supplements? • Does the coach encourage proper hydration during practices and games?

Many of the charts and checklists in this chapter can be printed out at
www.RealAge.com/parenting

Chapter 4

SPIFF UP
Convincing Kids That
Being Clean—Teeth to Toes—
Is Worth the Effort
(hey, you might even get
them to floss)

My daughter touches everything she sees and then sticks her fingers in her mouth."

"My son wears the same socks for two days and thinks brushing his teeth is optional."

"My teen shares *everything* with her girlfriends."

Sound familiar?

Keeping kids clean and free from germs is high on the list of things parents worry about. Most feel like their children are magnets for every bug that comes along—and many are. With all the sniffles, sneezes, coughs, and rashes passed around in schools today, classrooms are virtually petri dishes for germs. Because germs spread through close contact, the fact that kids constantly rub elbows with each other and touch everything in sight makes them particularly vulnerable to infections.

> The average child gets five to nine colds each year.

Children typically get five to nine colds a year and pre-schoolers seem to be the most susceptible, probably because young kids are more likely to put things in their mouths and less likely to wash their hands frequently.

Itchy yet?

Understand the Enemy—Good Germs Versus Bad

The fight against germs is one battle where it's really important to understand the enemy. Then evaluate your children's current defenses and improve their habits.

First of all, *germ* is an umbrella term for a range of tiny living organisms (also called microbes) that includes bacteria, viruses, and fungi. Along with other funky microscopic creatures, some germs can cause illness or infection (see the chart on page 110 for a quick overview). But 95 percent of germs are harmless. In fact, most are on your kids' side, working hard to keep them in good health. For example, microbes in the intestinal tract help kids digest food, and regular exposure to other germs actually helps immunize them against certain diseases.

What Different Types of Germs Can Do

Type	Description	Illnesses They Can Cause
Bacteria	One-celled organisms that can live and reproduce in or outside of the body. They multiply by subdividing. Less than 1% of all bacteria cause illness, but when infectious bacteria enter the body, they reproduce rapidly.	Cavities; pneumonia; impetigo; ear infections; bacterial meningitis; sinus infections; strep throat; urinary tract infections
Viruses (responsible for most common childhood diseases)	The smallest of the microbes, viruses need to be in or on a living thing (plant, animal, or human) to grow and reproduce. They travel on air currents or in body fluids. Virus particles can survive on surfaces for days and only a few are needed to infect someone.	Colds and flu; pneumonia; mononucleosis; viral meningitis; most coughs and sore throats; warts; chickenpox; measles; polio
Fungi	These include yeasts, mushrooms, and molds. Unlike other plants, fungi don't draw nourishment from soil, water, and air. Instead, they feed on plants, people, and animals. They love damp, warm places.	Yeast infections, including some forms of diaper rash; athlete's foot; ringworm; oral thrush; fungal nail infections
Protozoa	These one-celled organisms love moisture and often spread diseases through water. Some are parasites and need to live in other organisms.	Intestinal infections leading to diarrhea, nausea, and belly pain (protozoa cause malaria and dysentery)
Helminths	Tiny parasitic animals, helminths include pinworms and tapeworms.	Intestinal infections

But we may be making things so clean that kids' immune systems aren't challenged enough to develop strong disease-resistance skills. In addition, the overuse of antibacterial products may be creating "superbugs," germs that are tougher to get rid of than in the past. That's why I suggest going back to basics—plain old soap and water. They're still the best line of defense against most bad germs.

What can your family do to keep the good germs around and the bad ones at bay?

Plan Against Invasion

It's impossible to eliminate harmful germs entirely, but remember that old saying, "An ounce of prevention is worth a pound of cure." It doesn't take a ton of effort to guard kids against many germs.

Good hygiene habits are the gatekeepers to good health, restricting access and helping the immune system to run smoothly. They are your child's first line of defense—which again, boils down to those four steps we first talked about in Chapter 1: identify, inform, instruct, and instill. (By the way, this prevention plan works for all age groups, so put your whole family on it.)

1. **Identify: Where do germs sneak in?**
   Luckily, germs are pretty predictable. Most like to hitch rides on people's hands, but others travel through the air in sneezes or coughs, or through bodily fluids like sweat, saliva, or blood. Their favorite entry points are the mouth, nose, eyes, and skin.

2. **Inform: Explain what happens when germs get inside their bodies**
   It's important for children to know why good hygiene is so vital to their health. The consequences of carelessness

SHORT-TERM EFFECTS OF BAD HYGIENE	LONG-TERM EFFECTS OF BAD HYGIENE
• Itchy skin, acne, rashes, infections • More colds and flu • Bad breath • Body odor • Social difficulties • Pinworm • Food poisoning	• Scars from rashes and acne • Depressed immune system, meaning more illnesses • Cavities, gum disease (gingivitis) • Risk of serious infections • Career difficulties/social isolation due to poor personal care

often aren't immediately obvious, so it can be tough for children—and even adults, for that matter—to see the connection. That's where you come in. Talk to your kids about how their body works. Explain that bad germs make them sick and good personal habits keep them healthy. Discuss both the short- and long-term effects of neglecting these habits.

3. **Instruct: Teach kids how to stop germs in their tracks**
Okay, now your children know the basics about how germs get inside them and why cleanliness is important. Next, they need to know the single most important way to stop germs from invading:

Wash those hands, wash those hands, wash those hands.

Think about how many times kids rub their eyes, touch their nose, or put their fingers in their mouth. That's how germs gain entry—unless they've been washed down the drain. So wash, wash, wash—after using the bathroom, before eating, after coughing and sneezing, after being near someone who's sick, after coming home from school or any public place.

Of course, hand washing isn't the *only* good hygiene

habit you'll need to teach your child, but it's the first. We'll go over the others later.

4. **Instill: Praise children's germ-fighting skills**

    Just as with any new habit, kids need gentle reminders and praise while good, clean behavior is being learned. Also, let them see you brushing and flossing before bed or soaping up your hands after a trip to the playground or the restroom. They'll quickly get the idea and, with luck, you won't constantly have to say, "Did you remember to wash your hands?"

Evaluating Your Child's Current Habits

It's time to take a look at how your kids are doing when it comes to their personal care routines.

  Let's start with hygiene habit number one—how often do your kids wash their hands?

Probably not enough. In addition to washing hands when they are visibly dirty, children should always wash their hands:

BEFORE handling food or drinks, eating anything, taking medications, or putting on an adhesive bandage

AFTER using the bathroom, coming in contact with any body fluids (blood, sweat, urine, or vomit), coughing or sneezing, touching animals or pets, and administering first aid.

Is Antibacterial Soap Better? Do Sanitizer Gels Work?

Study after study has found that it doesn't matter what kind of soap you use. It's the sudsy rub-a-dub-dubbing that eliminates

Six Steps to Clean Hands

One in three boys and one in five girls don't wash their hands after using the restroom. A quick rinse doesn't count. Teach them how to do it right:

1. Wet hands with warm water.
2. Use enough soap to form a visible lather.
3. Scrub backs and fronts of hands, between fingers and under nails for at least fifteen seconds (the time it takes to recite the alphabet or sing "Happy Birthday").
4. Rinse well in warm, running water.
5. Dry thoroughly with a clean towel.
6. In public restrooms, turn off the faucet using a paper towel—lots of germs lurk on faucets.

germs. As for antibacterial soaps, there has been some debate over whether they produce resistant germs. The research isn't definitive, but the potential is there. For this reason, I think regular soap and water is just fine when it comes to everyday use.

When you're unable to get to a sink, alcohol-based hand sanitizers are a reasonable substitute. New research shows that these gels reduce the spread of germs around the house. In one study, families who used them cut the spread of gastrointestinal illness among family members by more than half. Kids can rub these gels on their hands and just let them air dry. Choose products containing at least 60 percent alcohol (listed on the label as isopropyl, ethanol, or n-proponal). Just be careful not to overuse these cleansers, as they can be very drying.

The Right Way to Cover Coughs and Sneezes

Here's another way germs get transferred: when kids cover their mouths as they cough or sneeze. It may seem like the polite thing to do, but coughing or sneezing into their hands spreads those germs onto everything their hands touch afterward—doorknobs, toys, books, softballs, other people. Anyone who touches one of those contaminated surfaces can get sick, too.

So here's a better method: Teach your child to turn away from people and cough or sneeze into a tissue or the crook of an elbow, pressing the mouth firmly into the arm. That way the germs are contained, minimizing the risk of spreading them.

Dental Care

Dental care is vital to health, so spend a lot of time on it. As soon as a child can hold a toothbrush, get started on brushing at least twice a day.

> *RealAge Projection:* Regular brushing and flossing are healthy habits no child can afford to skip. In fact, kids who stick with daily flossing and brushing in adulthood can shave as much as 6.4 years off their age. Their RealAge will still be in their early 30s when they're turning 40.

 ### No Teeth Yet?

Even infants need oral care. Take a clean wet cloth or gauze pad and gently wipe their gums and tongue after feedings to remove any bacteria and excess sugar that may have built up. As soon as the first tooth appears, brush gently with a soft, infant-sized toothbrush and plain water. Hold off on fluoride toothpaste until kids are old enough to spit it out—usually around age 3. Then use only a pea-sized dab. Try not to let kids swallow the toothpaste—and definitely don't let them eat

Avoiding Baby Bottle Tooth Decay

Tooth decay is a major issue for infants and toddlers because so much of what they drink contains sugar. And when a child slowly sucks on a bottle, the sugar lingers in the mouth, where oral bacteria turn it into an acid that eats away at tooth enamel.

You can avoid this by limiting bottles to mealtimes, and not letting kids fall asleep with a bottle in their mouth. For older children, quench late-night thirst with water. Also, encourage youngsters to start drinking from a cup around age 1; when a child drinks from a cup, the sugar moves past the teeth very quickly and does less harm.

Toothbrushing Tips

How much toothpaste: Although ads show a big S-shaped squirt, all kids need is a dab.
How long: Brush for at least two minutes, although dentists generally prefer three–four minutes.
Reality check: Most people spend only thirty seconds brushing.

Try using a three-minute egg timer to measure brushing time. Or find one of your kid's favorite songs that's about three minutes long and play it while they're brushing.

it out of the tube—as excess fluoride can be harmful.

 ### Brushing Baby Teeth

Make sure little kids have plenty of opportunities to watch you brush and ask them to "help" you brush your teeth. Kids are much more inclined to let you "have a turn" with brushing *their* teeth after they have first tried it on you. Young ones will probably need your help until age 5 or 6, but then should start brushing on their own; however, watch to be sure every tooth is reached, especially the back molars. Remember, twice a day is a minimum recommendation—if possible, encourage your child to brush after snacks, too, especially after sugary treats.

If you think brushing isn't all that important until permanent teeth come in, think again. Baby teeth are more susceptible to tooth decay than adult teeth, and even though they'll fall out, cavities can speed up this process and leave gaps. The remaining teeth may then shift to fill in the gaps—and cause the permanent teeth to come in crooked. Besides, if good brushing habits aren't established early, it's harder to get older kids to brush often and regularly.

Establishing good brushing habits early will help stave off tooth decay and gum diseases later, since many adults' oral health problems can be traced to poor childhood habits.

How to Make 'Em Brush More

One way to motivate kids to brush is to let them pick out their own toothbrushes and toothpaste. For toothbrushes, anything goes—from Barbie to zebra stripes—as long as they have soft bristles and are small enough to fit comfortably in a child-sized mouth.

Kids' toothpastes come in fun flavors and colors, too, such as bubble gum and Barney purple. Again, anything is fine, as long as it contains fluoride. Fluoride fights decay by making tooth enamel more resistant to bacteria. It has played a huge role in decreasing cavities among children.

Keep It Clean

A cluster of damp toothbrushes in the family bathroom can contribute to the spread of bacteria. Replace toothbrushes after any illness and at least every three months—the bristles wear out. Also, remind children to:

- Wash their hands before brushing
- Rinse the bristles thoroughly after use
- Shake any extra moisture from their brush
- Store it upright
- Never share toothbrushes

However, ingesting too much fluoride can cause fluorosis, a condition in which brown spots appear on children's teeth. The primary way children get too much is by swallowing fluoride rinses or fluoride toothpaste, especially with the tempting new toothpaste flavors out there. Although it takes a fair amount to be dangerous, be cautious (especially if your city's water supply is fluoridated, as most in the United States are).

Keep young children away from mouthwash. Because it usually contains alcohol—up to 30 percent—mouthwash ingestion by small kids can be dangerous, even lethal.

If your community's water is not fluoridated, or your kids drink bottled water exclusively, they either should take fluoride supplements—which a doctor or dentist can prescribe—or drink bottled water with added fluoride (check labels), beginning at 6 months.

Flossing

Unfortunately, brushing alone can't take care of the bad bacteria that live in the plaque between your child's teeth. Starting around age 3, or once most of the twenty primary teeth are in place, add daily flossing to the routine. You'll need to help kids with this until they're about 9 and have the hand skills to manipulate floss.

Why Flossing's Vital

Allowing the soft, sticky bacterial film called plaque to build up between the teeth invites all kinds of mouth trouble, including:

- Damaged enamel and decay
- Irritated, bleeding gums
- Smelly breath
- Tooth loss
- In severe cases, damage to the bone structure supporting the teeth

Don't be fooled into thinking that proper dental care is merely cosmetic, or even just about teeth and gums. It can have a much larger effect on overall health. Research has shown a distinct connection between serious oral health problems and cardiovascular disease in adults—it appears that bacteria from the mouth can enter the bloodstream and contribute to inflammation and artery clogging. **So keeping your child's mouth healthy now may keep his heart healthy later.**

Threaded flossers with a handle are easier for children to use than wrapping floss around fingers. Some come in fun shapes and bright colors, which can help get kids in the flossing habit.

Visiting the Dentist

If you have anxieties about visiting the dentist, try not to pass them on to your children. Seek out a dentist who enjoys working with children or specializes in pediatric dental care, has a kid-friendly waiting room, and maybe even offers little rewards—stickers, small toys, and the like—after a checkup. Kids who develop a good relationship with the dentist are likely to feel comfortable about getting regular cleanings and checkups. Routine dental exams uncover problems early, when repairs will be small, which helps eliminate the major, uncomfortable procedures that can make people develop a lifelong fear of dentists.

 ### Teens and Teeth

Ideally, teenagers already have well-established dental habits, but it's difficult to be sure because they usually shut the bathroom door. If you can't watch them brush, you can still talk about how important it is, especially if they have braces. Dire health warnings will likely fall on deaf ears, but try explaining that brushing and flossing twice a day helps:

> **Why Brush Before Bed?**
>
> To eliminate *Streptococci mutans*. These oral germs feed on sugar and cause tooth decay. They can multiply up to thirty times overnight.

- Keep you kissable—no dragon breath!
- Keep food from rotting between your teeth

- Keep staining and ugly tartar from darkening your smile
- Prevent dental visits that feature shots and drilling

If you have a battle over flossing in your house, keep mouth-wash around. It isn't a substitute for flossing, but it may help keep teen gums healthier. Their teeth are permanent now, so there are no do-overs.

Keeping Germs Out of the Mouth

Let's move on to other mouth issues, from "binkies" to nail biting.

 ### Babies Explore with Their Mouths

Well before kids begin brushing and flossing, they are busy put-ting things in their mouths. It's one of the main ways infants and toddlers explore their world. Although normal, this "mouthing" phase can definitely increase the number of microorganisms a child comes in contact with. But since you'd go bonkers trying to inspect and disinfect everything kids put in their mouths, focus on keeping the most popular items—pacifiers, teething rings, hands—as clean as possible.

Smart Pacifier Use

Binkies, ninnies, pacies, or dummies—whatever you call them, they're synonymous with babies. They fulfill the strong, instinc-tual urge to suck, and they give kids a way to self-soothe. But there are some guidelines to using them. First, don't use Mag-gie Simpson as a role model! A pacifier shouldn't be a constant fixture on your child's face. Research suggests that continuous sucking on a pacifier can contribute to bacteria moving from the throat to the middle ear, causing infections.

Try using pacifiers only for naps and at bedtime, to soothe your baby to sleep. Some studies show that limiting use in this way may help reduce the occurrence of ear infections.

It's a good idea to wean kids off pacifiers by age 1. Beyond this age, it can be a hard habit to break and may affect speech and dental development. You may have heard of many different ways to break the binkie habit, but as far as I'm concerned, nothing beats the cold-turkey approach. You may have to endure a day or two of whining, but stay strong. It'll soon be forgotten.

Pacifier Basics

Hold off on introducing a pacifier until your baby is 1 month old, so as not to interfere with breastfeeding. (Some babies don't seem to want to suck on a pacifier or their thumb, by the way, and that's fine. Don't push it.)

- Choose one-piece pacifiers that can't separate and become a choking hazard.
- Before using a new pacifier, soak it in boiling water or run it through the dishwasher.
- Don't "rinse" the pacifier in your own mouth; you'll just add more germs.
- Watch pacifiers for signs of deterioration and replace often.
- To prevent gum or tooth problems, never dip a pacifier in sugary liquids before offering it to a child. Also, don't place honey on pacifiers, as this common teething remedy can cause botulism.
- Never tie a pacifier on a cord and loop it around a baby's neck, or around a button or snap—the baby could strangle or choke on the cord.

Putting Babies Safely to Sleep

Although the cause of SIDS (sudden infant death syndrome) is still unknown, real progress has been made in preventing the unexplained, heartbreaking deaths of sleeping infants. In addition to taking the following precautions, encourage tummy time when babies are awake.

- Babies are much safer sleeping on backs, so never put infants under age 1 on their tummies to sleep, even for a quick nap.
- Recent research suggests that babies under age 1 who sleep with pacifiers have a reduced risk of sudden infant death syndrome (SIDS).
- Soft bedding can easily obstruct breathing, adding to the risk. Take pillows, stuffed toys, downy quilts, soft crib bumpers, and fluffy blankets out of the crib before putting a baby to sleep in it.
- Don't allow smoking anywhere near the baby (meaning anywhere in the home).
- Don't let infants share a bed with other children (or adults).
- Keep the room at a comfortable temperature for adults and dress your baby in light sleep clothing; overheating is a concern.
- If a blanket is needed, put the baby on its back with its feet almost touching the short end of the crib, place the blanket across the baby's chest (no higher) and tuck the edges under the mattress—or simply use a baby sleep sack.
- Never put a blanket over a baby's face or head.

Note that while SIDS can happen up to age 1, most deaths occur between 2 and 4 months, and the babies of certain ethnic groups are particularly vulnerable: African Americans, Native Americans, and Alaskan natives.

Teething Rings

Starting around 4 to 6 months, babies turn into little drool machines and begin gnawing on any hard object they can find. Although the eruption of teeth can be uncomfortable, avoid giving them pain-numbing gels or medications. Instead, gently rub their gums with a clean finger or, better yet, provide a cold teething ring or wet washcloth to bite on. Here's a trick that often works: Dip the corner of a washcloth in water and stick it in the freezer. Many babies love the icy spot's soothing/numbing effect. For really bad teething pain, a doctor may suggest children's Tylenol.

The steady flow of drool and saliva can cause rashes on the face and neck, so wipe your baby's face often with a soft, clean cloth. You also can rub a mild face balm on the cheeks and chin to protect them from drool. Placing a small, flat "drool cloth" under the baby's head in the crib will save you from having to change drool-covered sheets all the time. Just be sure that it, and anything you place in the crib, can't get loose or bunch up, creating a risk of asphyxiation.

> **Three Teething-Ring Tips**
>
> 1. The ring should be made of one piece of firm rubber.
> 2. Chill or freeze the ring for extra relief.
> 3. Check labels on teething rings filled with liquid—they should contain only distilled or purified water, just in case they break open.

Thumb Sucking

Many babies, toddlers, and even small children suck their thumbs or fingers. Don't worry. This is a perfectly normal childhood habit and quite soothing when kids are tired, upset, or bored. Just insist that they wash their hands often.

For most kids, thumb sucking usually fades away by age 5. However, if it is still going on when permanent teeth are coming in, it may cause problems. Children who suck their thumbs often have front teeth that stick out, requiring braces. Also, thumb sucking in school-age children can draw a great deal of teasing from other kids.

There are many ways to help a child who wants to kick

this habit but can't, such as putting bitter-tasting liquids on the thumb or wearing a finger-splint to bed. But one of the simplest ways is to have the child wear gloves for a few days. (This trick can also come in handy if you have a nail biter in the house.)

True Parenting Story: How Corey Broke Her Thumb-Sucking Habit

Our daughter Corey had just turned 4 and had started preschool, but she still sucked her thumb. I could tell she was ready to quit because she seemed very self-conscious about it, often hiding her face in the crook of her elbow when she did it. At first we tried to distract her whenever we noticed her thumb heading for her mouth and engage her in some activity that required both hands. Although this weakened the habit, it didn't stop it.

So we brainstormed with Corey and came up with the idea of creating a progress chart. Together we figured out what a reasonable number of "slip-ups" would be for each week and then tracked them with stickers on a poster board chart. We gave her a small prize at the end of each week she stayed within the limits—which got smaller and smaller—and then a larger reward when, at the end of five weeks, she kicked the habit. It worked like a charm.

We helped her along by putting an adhesive bandage on her thumb, especially at night, as a reminder. I'd heard about other methods, but luckily, the simple bandage did the trick.

—CAROL, WILTON, CT

  Nail Biting

Some young kids move straight from thumb sucking to nail biting. Others pick up the habit during adolescence as a way of coping with stress, and almost half of all adolescents and teens bite their nails to some degree.

The red, sore fingertips and bleeding cuticles that result invite infections around the nail beds. On top of that, kids touch countless germ-laden surfaces every day, and biting their nails allows germs easy access to the body. Long-term nail biting also can cause permanent nail damage and a deformed appearance. Sometimes it even leads to dental problems.

Children are more likely to stop biting their nails when they understand what triggers it. That means you first need to help them figure out the reason. Is it absent-minded biting—something done while absorbed in a book or watching TV? Or is it a sign of frustration, boredom, or stress? If so, help them find another way to cope—for example, squeezing a stress ball. The same tactics used to stop thumb sucking also can help kids kick the nail-biting habit.

> **How to Help Kids Quit Gnawing Their Nails**
>
> - **Point it out.** Gently remind them whenever the fingers go into the mouth.
> - **Treat the cause.** If the nail biting is stress related, work on stress-management techniques such as deep breathing, exercising, or meditation.
> - **Find a replacement.** Give kids something else to keep their hands busy when they start biting—even just doodling on a pad of paper or squeezing Silly Putty.
> - **Clip and trim.** Keep their nails as clean, trimmed, and filed as possible. If they look even somewhat nicer, kids may take better care of them.

Being Careful with Food

Bacteria can hitch a ride into your child's system through food. Salmonella, E. coli, and Listeria are just a few of the hundreds of organisms that can put kids at risk of food-borne illness, nausea, and diarrhea. Let kids know that it's hard to tell if food has been contaminated since germs often don't make food smell or taste bad. Explain that's why proper food handling—washing, cooking, refrigeration—is so vital. Above all, teach kids the importance of lathering up before digging in.

What About the Five-Second Rule?

Is food that has been on the floor fewer than five seconds safe for kids to eat? Generally speaking, no. It doesn't matter how quickly you pick it up. If the food lands where bacteria are, it will become contaminated almost immediately.

Shaking or blowing on the dropped food won't help. You may remove visible dirt, but the microscopic bugs aren't going anywhere.

I know many parents look the other way when their kids institute the five-second rule, and on occasion, I don't think this is anything to be really concerned about. But try not to let your kids make it a habit.

And of course, when in doubt, throw it out.

How Clean Is Your Kitchen?

Although many people believe they keep a clean kitchen, when videotaped while preparing meals at home, most adults made many food-handling mistakes that upped the risk of food-borne illness. Teach kids these basics, and be sure you practice them yourself!

- Always wash hands not only before eating or preparing food, but also between handling different foods, especially raw meat, poultry, and fish.
- Keep the food preparation area clean.
- Handle raw and cooked foods on separate work areas with separate cutting boards, knives, spoons, and other utensils.
- Wash all food that will be eaten raw (such as fruit and vegetables).
- Store foods at the correct temperature.

Protecting Your Child's Skin

Skin protects the body from exposure to harmful irritants and disease-causing germs. It is also home to a rich collection of microorganisms that play an essential balancing role in the body. These harmless bacteria are known as resident germs, and they guard against harmful transient bacteria that might otherwise take up residence there.

Don't forget to clean the cleaners and dryers. As a general rule, germs love moisture, so sponges, loofahs, and washcloths should all be cleaned, rinsed, and allowed to dry completely between uses to inhibit germ growth. Be sure to replace sponges and loofahs often, and clean your washcloths and towels with bleach or a bleach alternative, using the hottest setting of your washing machine.

 ### Bathing Baby

You can begin giving infants tub baths right away, but it is not necessary to bathe them daily. As long as they're changed and cleaned regularly in the diaper area—and around the ears and under the chin, where dribbles collect—they shouldn't need to be bathed more than every three or four days.

For young babies, small, plastic, infant bathtubs are safer than a full-size tub. Months later, when babies can sit on their own, they can graduate to the bigger tub. Either way, *never* leave babies unattended in the bath—tragedy can strike in just a few inches of water and a matter of moments.

Two Hints for Babies Who Don't Like Baths

- **Give them something to play with.** At first, this might be something as simple as a clean washcloth to suck on during the bath. Later, plastic cups make excellent pouring toys. Rubber dolls can also help them feel more comfortable. Blowing bubbles works magic for many kids.
- **Make silly hair sculptures.** While shampooing, make horns and shapes of all kinds with the soapsuds. Keep a hand mirror in the bathroom to show them the funny hairdos.

Go easy on the soap, which can cause dry skin. A gentle moisture-rich, liquid cleanser (such as Johnson's Baby Wash, Cetaphil, or Dove) is a good choice. Once out of the tub, lightly pat dry, leaving the skin a little damp, and immediately apply a cream or lotion to lock in the moisture.

 Time for Your Bath

Some kids are going to love to hear this: "Squeaky clean" is not always good. Although frequent bathing has aesthetic and stress-relieving benefits, it plays a minor role in disease prevention. In addition, some children have sensitive skin that may react badly to being bathed too often. For example, it can aggravate eczema, an irritating skin condition that causes itching. And the more kids scratch, the more irritated the skin becomes, increasing the chances of skin infections such as impetigo.

A daily bath is fine, but be sure to apply moisturizer right afterward; some kids may tolerate being fully bathed only once or twice a week, with sponge baths on the other days.

- Light sponging can be just as good as forceful scrubbing and it's less drying.
- Teach kids to focus on moist areas, such as the spaces between the toes, the groin, and the armpits, where germs can feed on sweat, oil, and cell debris.
- After washing, always pat skin dry instead of rubbing away.

 Teen Clean

It's one thing to worry about protecting young children from germs that can make them sick, but teenagers are a completely different animal. And there's so much more to worry about! You can't be there 24/7 to remind them to wash their hands, much less make sure they're wearing flip-flops in the locker room or not borrowing a friend's mascara. Plus, you have the usual hygiene concerns—from acne to body odor—and new worries as well, like do-it-yourself piercings, which can cause serious infections.

So what's the parent of a teen to do? Use the same method we've been talking about throughout this book: *Identify, inform, instruct,* and *instill* those good habits, and trust that your teenager will follow through. There's no guarantee that teens will practice good hygiene 100 percent of the time, but if your voice resonates in their head, they're more likely to make good choices. So discuss the following topics together.

Hit the Showers

Teens are famous for taking long, hot showers, but these are hard on their skin. Aim for five to ten minutes at most, using warm, not hot, water—and once a day is plenty. More frequent bathing will strip the natural oils from the skin, leaving it dry and irritated. For kids with busy sports schedules, encourage showers after they come home from sweat-inducing practices or games.

Genital Cleansing

Especially after puberty, remind tweens and teens how important it is to keep their entire bodies clean. Teenage boys and girls should bathe at least several times a week, clean genital areas with soap and water, and dry themselves off thoroughly in order to prevent infections.

Please, warn your daughter about the dangers of douching. While many women, young and old, use douches to feel more "clean," the truth is that douching puts them at risk for many different vaginal infections. It disrupts the natural balance of good organisms within the vagina that are responsible for keeping the area clean.

Hormones, Acne, and Body Odor

Changes in your child's smell are often the first indicator that puberty has begun. When you begin noticing that your son or daughter has a different sort of odor after returning from soccer practice, it's time to introduce deodorant. Neutralizing smell and sweat stains is important to self-esteem and peer acceptance, so encourage daily antiperspirant use.

Another issue brought about by puberty's hormonal changes is acne, which can have a devastating effect on self-image. For most kids, washing twice daily with a gentle facial cleanser and using over-the-counter acne medications is sufficient. Just discourage overwashing or hard scrubbing; both can actually increase oil production and exacerbate any problems. All cosmetics and lotions used on the face should be oil-free. For severe acne, prescription treatments are available; talk to the doctor about these.

Fungus Among Us

 Diaper Rash or Yeast Infection?

You might instantly think locker-room showers when you think of contracting a fungus, but even babies are at risk.

Candida, for example, is a type of fungus (commonly known

as a yeast infection) that can affect infants. It usually appears as a form of diaper rash, though it can also develop on other parts of a child's body, especially warm, moist areas such as a baby's neck. It starts as tiny red spots that multiply into a bright or dark red rash with distinct borders. If your baby is breastfeeding, sometimes the mother's breast becomes infected, too; yeast can also take up residence in the skin around the nails. Both mother and baby need to be treated to prevent reinfection.

 Sharing Tinea with Friends

Tinea, another type of fungal infection, is common among young kids and adolescents and is caused by several different types of fungus. It appears as a scaly rash, dry or moist, in many areas of the body, including the scalp, groin, hands, and feet. On the body, it usually appears as one or more coin-sized patches with a scaly ring and a smooth center. On the scalp, the rash is usually ringless and looks more like a scaly or bald spot.

Tinea spreads easily through contact with anything that has touched infected skin, which is why kids who love to share—trading combs, clothing, even shoes—are most susceptible. This is one instance when you want to discourage sharing.

Preventing Fungal Infections

Keeping skin clean and dry is the best defense against fungal infections. But kids are also less likely to get such infections by:

- Changing their socks and underwear every day
- Wearing airy, breathable clothing in warm weather
- Taking off their shoes at home and airing out their feet
- Throwing away grungy, worn-out exercise shoes
- Never borrowing someone else's shoes

Regularly check pets for areas of hair loss, which may signal a fungal infection. Your veterinarian can determine if this is a problem

Caution: Infections!

Most of the time, bacteria inhabit your children's skin without causing any problems. But if kids get a cut, scrape, or even an insect bite, everyday bacteria, such as *Streptococcus* and *Staphylococcus,* may begin to multiply and infiltrate tissue, causing a skin infection. The most common are cellulitis, folliculitis, and impetigo.

 Impetigo

Impetigo is a bacterial skin infection that typically affects school-age children in warm, humid weather. It causes a collection of small blisters or sores that may burst, ooze fluid, and develop a honey-colored crust. Outbreaks most frequently occur around the nose and mouth, but impetigo can appear anywhere and has a special preference for skin that is already

---

Locker Room Dos and Don'ts

Some terribly infectious things can grow in school locker rooms, showers, and pools. These warm, damp places provide ideal homes for many types of bacteria and fungi.

To help prevent jock itch, plantar warts, athlete's foot, ringworm, and other fungal infections, give teens these guidelines for showering and changing in the locker room.

- DO dry off thoroughly, especially between the toes, with a clean towel.
- DON'T share towels with anyone.
- DO wear shower shoes or sandals everywhere (yes, in the shower).
- DON'T sit on shared benches, especially if they're damp—these are havens for germs.
- DO spray lockers weekly with a disinfectant spray.

irritated from, say, eczema, poison ivy, insect bites, or a reaction to soap. Impetigo is very contagious—touch it with the fingers and it spreads easily to other areas of the body, and it also spreads to other household members on towels, clothing, and bed linens that touched the person's infected skin. Your doctor will treat it with antibiotics.

Cleaning Scrapes and Scratches

Carefully cleaning cuts and abrasions as soon as possible after the injury occurs reduces the risk of infections and scarring. Wash all new wounds gently but thoroughly with soap and running water for five to ten minutes. Because puncture wounds are more likely to become infected, soak these injuries in soapy water for fifteen minutes (and be sure tetanus shots are up to date; punctures are often caused by rusty or dirty metal objects). Antibiotic creams and ointments will help keep the tissue moist and fight bacterial invasion. A bandage can help keep germs out, but don't make it too tight and change it daily—or immediately if it becomes dirty or wet.

Clear Signs of a Skin Infection

Please seek medical attention if any of these symptoms occur:

- Wound becomes very tender
- Pain or swelling increases forty-eight hours after the initial injury
- Wound oozes pus or fluid
- A yellow crust forms on the wound
- Scab size increases, rather than decreases
- Redness increases around the wound (cellulitis)
- A red streak spreads outward from the wound
- The wound isn't healed within ten days
- The child develops a fever over 100°F

  Could I Borrow Your Conjunctivitis?

Young kids, tweens, and teens are notorious for sharing pretty much anything—toys, hairbands, makeup, sports gear, you name it—and this can spread various bacterial and viral infections, including conjunctivitis, or pinkeye.

Conjunctivitis is a highly contagious eye infection that causes redness, itching, and discharge. Avoiding it means (a) trying to keep small hands out of infected eyes; (b) for teens, *never* sharing eye makeup with friends; and (c) for kids who wear contact lenses, being rigorous about keeping them clean (see box).

 Infections from Body Piercings and Tattoos

Once, the only piercing-related infections I saw were on earlobes. Today, teens pierce their noses, eyebrows, navels, tongues, and more. Many of these are infection-prone areas, especially if the piercings aren't done in a sanitary manner. Tattoos, even if done by a professional, can also lead to serious infections and even diseases.

Because many states require parental permission for piercings and tattoos for kids under 18, many teens try to do it themselves, which can be quite dangerous. Home piercings can cause severe infections, excessive bleeding, and even nerve damage. Home tattoos can lead to bacterial, fungal, and viral infections—including hepatitis and HIV—and can cause allergic reactions, toxic shock syndrome, tetanus, and skin diseases.

Talk to your teens about the risks. If you wind up agreeing to these forms of self-expression, be sure they're done by a reputable piercer or tattoo artist who uses sterile tools.

Critters to Consider: How to Shoo Those Little Buggers Away

No matter how clean your kids are, it may be next to impossible to avoid some common nuisances, like head lice and pinworms—nearly every child has to deal with at least one of these at some point. Still, there are ways to reduce the risk, and if you teach your children well they may just be one of the lucky few.

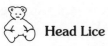 **Head Lice**

These tiny, wingless parasitic insects live in kids' hair and feed on small amounts of blood drawn from the scalp. Outbreaks are especially common among kids 3 to 12 since this age group tends to have close physical contact and often shares things. Contact is the only way to pass lice on to another person, and they move quickly! Remind kids not to share *any* items that come in contact with their heads—combs, brushes, hats, scarves, bandanas, ribbons, barrettes, hair ties, headbands, towels, and helmets.

> **Home Remedy for Lice**
>
> Soak the hair and scalp with Cetaphil liquid cleanser; comb out the excess and use a hair dryer to dry the lotion in place. Leave it on long enough to suffocate the lice—at least eight hours—then wash it out.

If your child does become infected, you'll see tiny pearly white ovals called nits, which are lice eggs, attached to hair strands about ½ inch from the scalp. You may also see lice, which are small brown insects. The first line of attack is over-the-counter lice-killers (Rid, Nix), but there are now resistant strains that respond only to prescription treatments. There are also some home remedies—their shared premise is to suffocate the lice—that many people swear by. If you want to try

Delousing Your House

Once one person in the family has head lice, you'll need to go all out to keep everyone else in the house from getting them. Here's what to do.

- Wash all clothing, towels, and bed linens in hot water and then dry them on the hottest cycle for at least twenty minutes.
- Dry clean anything else—plush toys and pillows, too—that can't be machine-washed, or seal them in air-tight bags for one week.
- Thoroughly vacuum all rugs, carpeting, upholstered furniture, car seats, and floor mats.
- Soak combs, barrettes, headbands, brushes, and all other hair items in rubbing alcohol or medicated shampoo for one hour—run them through the dishwasher or just throw them away.

one of these, putting mayonnaise in the hair is messy but does seem to work, as does coating the hair with Cetaphil, a gentle skin cleanser (see box, page 135). But the only surefire way to eradicate these critters is to meticulously comb through your child's hair with a fine-tooth comb and pick out each little nit. Also, be on the lookout for the LouseBuster in 2008. This blow dryer-like device, which zaps lice and eggs with hot air, is currently in testing and the initial results look promising.

Pinworms

If your child wakes in the night, scratching his bottom and crying out for you to "Make it stop!" think pinworms. They're very common among kids. The small white worms, less than a half an inch long, take up residence in the intestines and lay their eggs around the anus, causing an itchy bottom, especially during the night.

Pinworms are very easy to get: The minuscule eggs are often picked up on hands while playing with other children; the hands touch the child's mouth; the eggs are swallowed and hatch in the upper intestine. The new female pinworms then lay their eggs near the anus. If the child scratches his itchy bottom, the eggs can get under his nails (where they can live for several hours) and be transferred to family members, playmates, and pretty much anything in the house. Pinworm eggs can live for weeks on clothes, toys, and bedding.

Most cases are diagnosed with a tape test: cellophane tape is pressed against the skin around the anus and then viewed by a doctor under a microscope to check for pinworm eggs.

Luckily, pinworms are fairly easy to treat. Over-the-counter and prescription medications are available. If one member of the family is infected, it's a good idea to treat the entire household, because pinworms are easily spread. In addition, wash all bedding, towels, plush toys, and clothing in hot water and keep everyone's fingernails extra-clean and cut short.

  ### Below the Belt—Avoiding UTIs

Another common problem for kids are urinary tract infections (UTIs). The usual symptoms are a frequent urge to urinate, difficulty doing it, and a burning sensation when they go. If your child says it hurts to pee, see the pediatrician for a urinalysis and culture to determine if it needs to be treated with a round of antibiotics. Call right away. These things can quickly get worse. Also, be aware that in young kids, frequent wetting accidents, day or night, can be a sign of a UTI.

Here's how UTIs get started. Bacteria live at the end of the urethra—the tube that empties urine

How to Prevent a UTI

Tell your children:

- Don't "hold it"—go to the bathroom as soon as the urge hits.
- Drink lots of fluids; going often helps.
- Relax and completely empty the bladder.
- Girls: Lower pants to the ankles and sit comfortably on the toilet, with feet on floor (or step stool).
- Girls: Wipe thoroughly from front to back. (Demonstrate on a doll.)
- Boys: Open pants and underpants completely so there's no pressure on the genitals.
- Thoroughly wash hands afterward with soap and water.

from the bladder—and on the skin around the opening of the urethra. When harmful bacteria find their way up the urethra and into the bladder, they can cause a UTI (or cystitis).

Girls tend to get UTIs more often because their urethras are shorter and closer to the anus, where troublesome bacteria—usually E. coli—lurk. Taking frequent bubble baths, using perfumed soaps or body washes, or improper wiping can irritate the urethra, and make urinary infections more likely.

Diligence, Discipline, and Patience

Germs are an unavoidable part of your child's world, and most are usually benign. But those that aren't can cause real problems if daily hygiene habits get a little lax. During the first couple of years, a lot of the responsibility for kids' cleanliness rests on your shoulders. However, everything you do, even in those first few weeks and months, lays the foundation for healthy future habits. And that's a major investment in your children's well-being for years to come.

Many of the charts and checklists in this chapter can be printed out at
www.RealAge.com/parenting

Chapter 5

SMARTEN UP
Teaching Kids Good Homework Habits
(the kind that will get them ahead in school)

Kids are like sponges. You've no doubt heard this comparison, and it's true. They soak up everything around them. When encouraged, they're superabsorbent. But if they're squeezed too hard (or not hard enough), they turn into soggy sponges, leaking tears of frustration.

The point is that all children learn differently. Some are visual learners while others are auditory learners. Some need lots of encouragement; others need to figure things out on their own. Either way, you want to help them make the most of their learning style.

But before you run off and sign up your child for tutoring or advanced classes, step back and find out what your kid really needs to succeed.

It might be discovering reading for fun and relaxation. It might be make-believe or music or art. Or study buddies and socialization. Identifying your child's strengths and weaknesses (there's always a mix) and figuring out ways to enhance both is an essential step in helping your child become a lifelong learner and achiever.

Your Child's Approach to Learning

When it comes to solving a new puzzle, playing a game, or doing homework, does your child do any of the following?

- Throw a fit
- Whine
- Procrastinate
- Become frustrated
- Cry easily
- Seem disinterested
- Become angry

Or does your child:

- Show effort and perseverance
- Take pleasure in success
- Express an eagerness to learn
- Express frustration appropriately

Parents are always curious about their child's intellectual capabilities and development. Is my child average? Below average? Gifted? Showing signs of a learning disability? Regardless of the answers, parents want reassurance that they are doing everything they can to encourage advancement.

Gifts Can Be a Challenge

Consider Jamie, a 7-year-old I saw, along with his parents, for what at first seemed like a routine checkup. I quickly realized that Jamie was exceptionally bright. His vocabulary was huge for a second grader, and when I asked about school, he described in great detail a science unit about magnets. His mother chimed in about the elaborate stories Jamie wrote, usually concerning robots, rocket ships, and outer space.

But Jamie's parents were concerned. Their son was prone to outbursts and crying at school. These episodes were not only a distraction in the classroom, but they were creating social problems for him as well. He was often teased on the playground, with a few of the boys calling him a "crybaby," which sparked even more tears.

It turned out that these outbursts had begun two years before when Jamie started kindergarten. I began to suspect that his emotional outcries were related to a lack of stimulation at school.

"He's always been ahead of the curve," Jamie's father explained. "I worry that he gets bored. He zips through his schoolwork so fast that he has a lot of extra time to fill." It was clear that Jamie wasn't being challenged, and because he already knew or quickly grasped the information taught to him, he didn't really feel like part of the class. Instead, he felt isolated and unaccepted by both his teacher and his peers.

Many children who are very academically advanced struggle socially. Their people skills are often not as advanced as their academic skills, and they have a hard time relating to their peers.

I suggested that Jamie's parents talk with his teacher about ways to accommodate his giftedness and get him more involved. If his school didn't have an accelerated-learning program, perhaps it was time to find one that did. (See the checklist at the end of this chapter for things to consider when picking a school for your child.) Jamie's parents could also help by finding after-school activities—a science club, for example—that would allow him to form friendships with children whose interests and abilities are more in line with his own.

"How far do we go? I mean, we want him to be challenged, but how do we know when it's too much? And how do we help him fit in?" Jamie's father asked.

Good questions. You may be facing similar issues, wondering how to ensure that your child is being challenged, without overdoing it. Plus you want your child to fit in and have friends.

Nurturing the Gifted Child

All children need validation and acceptance, and sometimes gifted kids may repress their intellectual ability, pretending they don't know as much as they really do so that they can fit in. Conversely, they can be boastful or know-it-alls, which often alienates their classmates.

A mentor can often help. If you can find one who is a good match for your child, the relationship can really help develop social skills and provide encouragement, inspiration, and insights as well. If your child is open to the idea, ask the teacher to help identify a few mentor candidates.

Uneven Development

Finally, gifted children are often perfectionists and set high standards that can create a lot of stress in their lives. Parents have their own expectations. Be careful not to convey a desire for perfection. Allow children to see you fail in everyday tasks like attempting a new recipe or a carpentry project. Help them to understand that learning is a process, that everything doesn't come easily, and that sometimes good enough is—good enough.

Learning Starts Very Early

From the time they are infants, kids are soaking up information about the world around them. Some soon-to-be parents try to get a head start by speaking, playing music, and reading to their baby long before birth! It may seem silly at first, but researchers have determined that cognitive development begins in the womb. Many factors in the prenatal environment, such as nutrition and hormones, can affect the early development of the skills that infants and children will use later. For example, children start learning about sounds before birth. Just how much they learn prenatally is not yet known, but starting early can't hurt.

Again and Again

As parents, you delight in your kids' milestones: first words, learning to read. But your kids wouldn't be making such intellectual progress on their own. You, along with the other significant people in their life, provide the stimulation essential for that growth. Talking, singing, and reading to your children develops connections in the brain that become stronger with time and repetition. A young child's brain is actually wired to encourage repetition of sounds, patterns, or experiences. This "echoing" provides a feeling of comfort and security, and develops strong neural pathways in the brain that become the highways of learning. That's why young children love to hear the same song or the same story over and over again.

Exasperating to parents? Yes. Important for a child's cognitive development? Absolutely! So take a deep breath, and get ready to sing "Wheels on the Bus" for the fifteenth time. It's helping your baby's brain develop.

Reading Really Is Fundamental

From the moment you know you're expecting, you dream of the life you want for your child. An artist? A teacher? A doctor? It doesn't matter, as long as you start your child down the path to success in school.

First off, reading to your children is the most significant way to encourage brain development. I can't emphasize this enough. Whether you're reading to your unborn baby (try to do this daily during the last trimester) or your baby (do this daily too), or turning pages with your toddler on the couch, or reading bedside before lights-out, it's a special time for you and your child. Not only does it strengthen your bond, but it associates reading with warm feelings, prompting them to want to read more.

> **Other Ways to Make Reading Fun:**
>
> - **Chat it up.** Talk about the story together.
> - **Mix it up.** Have your child come up with an alternate ending.
> - **Keep 'em guessing.** Ask your child to guess what will happen next.
> - **Involve them.** Discuss ways to deal with a challenge or problem in the story.
> - **Be dramatic.** Use different voices for each character in the story.
> - **Take turns.** Trade off reading chapters, once kids learn to read.

Even after kids learn to read on their own, it's still important to have read-aloud time together. Also, ask older children to read to younger siblings. They'll be proud, and the younger kids will be even more enthusiastic about learning to read.

The First Three Years and Beyond

Experts agree that a huge amount of cognitive development occurs before age 3. The neurological connections made then affect how children organize and coordinate information, how they reason, and how they solve problems. That means experiences in the first few years of life are crucial to future success in school and in life. So you really are your child's first and most important teacher!

The more language-rich you make your child's preschool environment, the better. By consistently asking questions, explaining answers, and just talking, you provide the stimulation your child needs. Children who are continually stimulated by language tend to score higher on intellectual tests.

Once in kindergarten, learning really starts to blossom. Most parents are awed by the growth of their children's intellect from the time they enter kindergarten to the time they graduate from it. They learn *so* much in such a short time.

But what about after kindergarten? Children's knowledge obviously continues to grow, but the milestones aren't as easy to pinpoint. That's why it's par-

Stay in Touch

Start off the school year by sending your child's teacher(s) a short letter introducing yourself. Also, fill out the checklist at the end of this chapter and include it in the letter. Follow up with quick updates throughout the school year, highlighting anything new that's going on with your child or at home. Some teachers even provide an e-mail address at which they can be contacted.

ticularly important to stay involved with your kid's intellectual development throughout their school years. Help with homework when needed, keep the lines of communication open with teachers, and attend PTA meetings and parent/teacher conferences.

Intellectual Milestones: What to Look For

At the end of this chapter, there's a checklist to help you track where your child is developmentally. However, remember that children develop at their own pace and it's next to impossible to predict exactly when a child will master a skill. Still, the following will give you a general idea of when changes tend to occur. Don't be alarmed if your child hasn't reached certain milestones for her age; just take note of it and look at the bigger intellectual picture. Chances are there isn't anything to worry about, but if you're concerned, bring it up at your child's next checkup.

Brain Gains: Evaluating Your Child's Intellectual Development

So how do you think you're doing when it comes to nurturing your child's brain? Obviously, the first three years of life are crucial, but your job as a cheerleader for learning doesn't end there. From birth to age 18 (and even beyond) you will encounter opportunities to help engage, challenge, and support your children so they can achieve their ultimate potential and attain success in and out of school.

Let's take a look at your answers to the RealAge Healthy Kids Test questions about learning, and perhaps you'll learn a little something as well.

How much sleep does your child get on most nights?
All children need plenty of sleep to function at their best. Kids who don't get enough sleep at night may find it hard to concentrate throughout the day, which will undermine their performance. Although every child is different when it comes to the need for sleep, there are general guidelines I suggest to parents. For children 9 and under, ten or more hours at night is optimum. For ages 10 and over, about nine and a half hours is best.

Enforce a bedtime that allows your child to get enough sleep. Not the easiest of tasks if you're the parent of a teenager who would rather stay up late and watch TV or instant message friends than get some extra shut-eye. That's why I recommend no TVs, computers, or video game players in the bedroom. Make it a place for sleep—not recreation. No doubt your teen will mumble and groan when you take this step, but it's important, especially if your child's grades aren't what they could be.

Bringing on the Sandman

What else can you do to ensure kids get enough sleep? The following suggestions may be adapted for an older or younger child. Just be aware that what's calming for one child can be stimulating to another, so you may need to experiment a bit:

- **Get stuck in a rut.** Establish a regular routine. Knowing what time the evening always ends reduces bedtime battles.
- **Fill the belly.** A small snack about an hour before bedtime can help quiet a rumbling tummy.
- **Have a soak.** A warm bath can be a soothing transition to sleep.
- **Set the mood.** Create a sleep-friendly environment for young kids: dimmed lighting, soft music, a favorite blanket or stuffed animal.
- **Stick with it.** Once you've set up a sleep routine, be consistent, even on weekends.

Identifying Sleep Disturbances

If your child is getting enough sleep and still seems tired, check for a medical problem. There are a few conditions that can disrupt sleep habits. Does your child frequently wake up at night—

either three or more times or for a total of at least an hour? A recent study found that nearly 20 percent of grade-school kids suffer from sleep disturbances such as these. Sleep apnea—a snoring, gasping condition—can occur when enlarged tonsils or adenoids block the airway. It's fairly common in kids and makes sleeping difficult. Trouble sleeping may also be a sign of an emotional problem, such as anxiety or depression. Work with your pediatrician to find the cause and solutions for sleep problems.

What is the total time per day your child spends watching TV or playing video games?

Too much TV and computer time isn't just bad for kids' bodies. It also seems to be bad for their brains.

New studies show that TV may actually alter the hardwiring in young brains, shortening attention spans and causing problems with focus and concentration. One study found that 1- to 3-year-olds who watched TV daily had more attention-related difficulties by age 7 than children who watched only occasionally. Not only that, the more TV they watched, the more problems they had.

I know some kids, especially teens, who swear they work better with the TV on. With few exceptions, I don't think that's true. The TV is distracting, plain and simple. As soon as kids get into the groove of a school assignment, a cool commercial for a favorite program comes on. They stop to watch, then it takes a few minutes to refocus on homework again—then something else on TV catches their attention. You get the picture.

What's the Right Amount?

Attention problems are not the only worry. Time spent in front of the tube is time *not* spent in more creative endeavors. Less than an hour a day of TV and video games is ideal, but try telling that to a 9-year-old Nintendo nut. Still, moderate how much your kids watch. New guidelines from the American Academy of Pediatrics (AAP) recommend *no* viewing time for children under 2, and no more than one or two hours a day of educational, nonviolent programs for older children. However, quality shows can have a positive effect on learning—preschoolers who watch them do better on reading and math tests, reports the AAP. In other words, the right amount of the right programming can be educational.

On the other hand, here's what kids see who watch three to four hours of noneducational TV a day: about 8,000 murders and 20,000 commercials a year. No kid needs that.

How about the computer? How much time does your child spend each day using it for things other than schoolwork?

Computers are great for learning about anything, and it's amazing to see how adept kids are at using them, researching school projects, joining online groups to chat about a favorite topic, even e-mailing their teachers. But like TV time, computer use for things other than schoolwork should be limited. Less than an hour of non-schoolwork time should be enough for most children.

The jury is still out on the effects of computer use on cognitive and social development. Some studies show that children who live in homes with a computer have slightly higher literary and math skills. The research on the social impact of computer use is a little fuzzier than that on heavy TV viewing. But clearly, if a child is spending hours a day on the computer, direct interaction with other kids is reduced. Chat rooms and instant messaging just aren't the same as face time. As a result, kids may not be learning the social skills they need.

Kid-safe Searching

These search engines are perfect for kids. They connect them only to sites that the editors have handpicked as appropriate for children. Any inappropriate sites are filtered out.

Ask Jeeves for Kids
www.ajkids.com

Kids Click!
www.kidsclick.org

LookSmart's Kids Directory
www.netnanny.com

Yahooligans!
www.yahooligans.com

Instill These Rules for Safe Surfing

- **Remain anonymous.** Don't give out personal info: name, birth date, address, city, school.
- **Go undercover.** Create an alias.
- **Raise red flags.** Alert an adult if inappropriate contact is made by someone in a chat room, on a bulletin board, or through e-mail.
- **Be nice.** No flaming, spamming, or bullying allowed.
- **No pictures.** Limit or prohibit posting photos on a personal Web page or online community.
- **No talking to strangers.** No opening e-mail from someone unknown.

Can playing violent computer or video games lead to violent or aggressive behavior?
There's research supporting both sides of that issue. Some studies suggest that children behave in a more aggressive manner after playing computer games with violent themes, but some don't. In my experience, the effects, if any, vary with the individual child. A kid who's already verging on the overaggressive might be encouraged to become more so by certain games, whereas one who's inherently gentle is unlikely to be changed.

My overall concerns—academic, social, and physical—with spending excessive amounts of time playing these games remain, however, regardless of whether they're fun or violent. If you're at all worried about the language or violence in a game your child wants, read the warnings on the box about the nature of the content. If you buy it, but hesitatingly, watch the game yourself with your child. Turn it off if you feel it's inappropriate and talk to your child about the content.

Is your child supervised (either by an adult or by software) when using the Internet?

If you answered no, decide to change it to yes. Your child should be supervised while using the Internet. While it offers all sorts of useful information, there's just as much that isn't kid-appropriate. Instead of letting your kids use general search engines such as Google or Yahoo, try more child-friendly ones that filter out the junk (see Searching box).

Obviously, it's not feasible to watch every moment that your child spends surfing the Web. Good reason to install a filter on the computer that will keep your child safe and allow you to track what sites are visited. It's also another reason to kick computers out of kids' bedrooms, where iffy late-night surfing is far more likely.

Set up house rules for using the computer, and teach kids safe and smart (and polite) online behavior (see Surfing box, page 150). It may help to post a set of guidelines in sight of the computer so they're reminded each time they sign on.

Does your child have a special area in the home that's specifically for doing homework?

The best place to do homework depends largely on your child's work style. Granted, some kids have trouble concentrating with even the slightest distraction—a

---

Help Kids "Get It" at School

Children are motivated not only by achieving success—an A on a paper or 95 percent on a math test—but also by understanding what they're learning. Kids want to "get it" and they have an innate desire to keep on trying, even if they fail at first.

Take riding a bike. I doubt if any child has learned to ride a bike without a few scratches and bruises along the way. But no matter how long it takes, they don't give up.

The elation kids feel once they're pedaling by themselves is akin to the feeling they get when they read their first book, or finally understand how to find the value of x in an algebra problem. That "aha!" feeling will keep them reaching for more—more successes, more knowledge, and more understanding of the world around them.

baby sister in the same room, for example. They should have a quiet place to work. For most kids, however, the perfect place for homework is at a kitchen or dining table, where they can easily ask you or other family members for help if they need it. This arrangement is good for you too, because it makes it easier to stay involved with what your child is learning and to recognize your child's strengths and struggles.

Of course, if your child is more comfortable sprawling on the floor—or for that matter, studying in a tree house—fine. Having a regular place to do homework will establish great study habits early on, and that's vital for overall success at school.

Try to have supplies readily available. It cuts down on time spent looking for a glue stick or a red marker, leaving the focus where it belongs: on homework. Restock as supplies run low—unless you enjoy running to the store just before it closes, hoping to find what you need. Here are a few suggestions:

- Paper: notebook, graph, construction, tracing, and computer
- Glue and glue sticks
- Tape
- Pens, pencils, crayons, markers
- Scissors
- Hole punch
- Calculator
- Ruler
- Report folders
- Poster board

When does your child do homework?

Setting a consistent homework time is another way to help establish good study habits. While some parents think it's best to wait until after dinner, I suggest that they start doing it within an hour after getting home from school. First, let your child take thirty or forty minutes to recharge, run around with the dog, have a snack, or chat with you, but then get it done. If you delay homework until after dinner, your child—and you—may be too tired to complete an assignment, especially one that's challenging. Things can turn cranky fast, leading to stress that can disrupt sleep.

If the only time available to do homework is after dinner and grades aren't suffering, work with that. But if every night leads to a battle, or grades have dropped, it might be time to cut back on extracurricular activities that interfere with getting schoolwork done.

Try to avoid letting your child finish homework in the morning before school, especially after a late night of studying—though it's better than not getting it done at all. Still, mornings should be focused on filling your child's belly with nutritious food for the day ahead, not finishing work that should have been completed the night before. If playing homework catch-up is a familiar scenario, ask yourself a few things:

- Is the amount of homework appropriate?
- Is your child struggling with the level of work assigned?
- Is your child leaving assignments until the last minute?

It's your child's responsibility to actually do the homework, but it's your responsibility to ensure that it's done. Establishing good homework habits when kids are young will make a huge difference as they grow older and begin coping independently with school assignments.

Should You Help Children with Their Homework?

The answer is yes, but only to a certain extent. Your children count on you to help explain connections between things that are new to them and what they already know. Be available for questions during homework time—supporting their efforts to grasp new material and reshaping information to fit their level of understanding.

Good Homework Help
- **Chop it up.** Break large projects down into smaller, more manageable components.
- **Go easy.** Start with the simple stuff. If kids start with the most difficult, they may be too tired or upset to complete the assignments that are a breeze.
- **Let them do it.** Don't give them the answers—help them find the answers.
- **Prioritize.** Ask them what they can do on their own and what they might need help with. Success with one task may make them suspect they can do the others, too.
- **Get organized.** Teach kids how to manage time with a notebook or calendar that tracks assignments and due dates.
- **Buddy up.** Set up study groups or phone meetings with a study buddy. Encourage older children to tutor younger siblings, or help in some way: quiz them on a spelling list, help construct a diorama, use multiplication flashcards.

How does your child spend leisure time?

We live in a technology-rich era. Electronic media is everywhere, entertaining us as well as influencing our choices. But it shouldn't take over our lives. Help your kids get back to basics by encouraging other forms of recreation, like reading, backyard games, or arts and crafts. You might be surprised to find out how much your children actually learn through unstructured play. Not only is it healthy for their bodies, but it's healthy for their minds.

Left to their own devices, kids have always managed to entertain themselves. You've likely witnessed a small child cast aside the shiny new toy in favor of the cool box it came in. Try to look at ordinary things—a plastic ice cube tray, an old steering wheel—with the eyes of a child. If these items don't present a safety hazard, add them to the toy box or leave them where your kid will find them. Provide an environment that encourages play and then step back and let the learning begin. A few more suggestions:

- Stock kids' shelves with blocks, art supplies, and dress-up clothes.
- Recycle plastic containers that can be used to hold water, pour sand, or hide secret treasures.
- Keep cardboard boxes: They might be perfect as a dollhouse, fire station, or barnyard corral.
- Reserve old blankets and pillows for making cozy tents, caves, and forts.
- Stash scarves and fabric remnants for make-believe costumes—a beautiful headdress or superhero cape.

The Educational Value of Games

Games are much more than just a way to exercise the body. They're also a great way to enhance the mind. They teach kids to self-regulate themselves—independently, they learn the value of rules and the consequences when rules are broken. For example, in a playground game everyone waits for a turn. If someone tries to cut in, someone might not get a turn. Kids quickly determine what is fair and what isn't. Rather than being told by an adult which rules to follow, they figure it out on their own.

Playing games also sharpens certain skills. For example, from plotting their next move in checkers, managing their money in Monopoly, and taking turns in Old Maid, kids learn strategy, logic, reasoning, and social skills.

Which clubs, activities, or organizations does your child participate in regularly?

This question is also discussed in Chapter 3, but here it's in the context of learning and intellectual development. After-school

Making Real-World Connections

What kids learn at school may not have a lasting impact if it seems unrelated to everyday life. But if they can quickly put new information to practical use, they're more likely to see how it can help them in the real world. Here are some ways parents can help link classroom learning to their kids' lives:

- Read the Sunday newspaper with tweens and teens. Discuss or debate local news or hot national topics. Doing so will help them develop critical-thinking skills.
- Talk about world events and how they relate to a middle-school child's history or geography class.
- With a budding mathlete, discuss the price of gas as a way to practice working with percentages.
- Let younger children use their own money to buy something they want, then talk about how much items cost and how much change they should receive.
- Dictate your grocery list to a child to improve writing skills.
- Cook together. Measuring recipe ingredients gives meaning to numbers and fractions.

activities should be an important part of every child's life. They let kids really dig into specific interests and demonstrate that learning isn't confined to classrooms. In addition, intellectually stimulating activities help keep kids' minds sharp by creating new brain cell connections. And if mind games such as chess, crosswords, and logic puzzles become an ongoing part of your child's life, it could help ward off certain types of dementia much further down the road.

RealAge Projection: **If children develop an appreciation for learning when they're young, they're likely to maintain a hunger for knowledge as they get older. If they do, when they turn 40, they'll be more like 37.**

Roadblocks to Success

All children stumble on the path of intellectual development, whether they're exceptionally bright or functioning below the norm. And some children also struggle with physical and behavioral challenges that hinder their ability to learn. These include hearing or speech problems, learning disorders such as dyslexia, and behavioral problems such as ADHD. These challenges occur more often than you may think, and it's critical to remain vigilant. If you suspect that there's a problem brewing—whether it's ADHD, dyslexia, not being strong in math, or being understimulated—discuss it with your child's teacher, school, and pediatrician. It's important to deal with problems as early as possible.

Basic Facts about ADHD

Attention deficit hyperactivity disorder, or ADHD, makes learning difficult for many children. As many as 3 to 5 percent of kids in the United States have it, so chances are good that every classroom has at least one child struggling with ADHD.

ADHD is a biological disorder, not just bad behavior. The symptoms often mirror normal childhood behavior—exuberance, boundless energy, and lots of rapid-fire questions—but taken to such an extreme that it impairs kids' ability to function in daily life. How can you recognize a kid with the disorder? Children with ADHD have three main symptoms:

1. They have serious difficulty paying attention.
2. They are *very* active.
3. They are often very impulsive.

Three different types of ADHD have been found to affect both children and adults:

1. Inattentive—real difficulty focusing on tasks
2. Hyperactive-Impulsive—very busy, and often act before thinking
3. Combined—inattentive, hyperactive, and impulsive

A Mother's Concern about ADHD

Matthew, an active 7-year-old, and his mother, Judy, came to see me. From the moment Judy began talking, I noticed tears welling up in her eyes.

"Matthew's school evaluated him for attention problems, and asked me to talk to you about their findings," she said, handing me the school's assessment report. "His teacher mentioned that he might need to take medication. That really worries me because of all I've heard about the overmedication of children these days. I don't want to put him on drugs if it's not absolutely necessary."

The report listed all the tests given to Matthew to assess his behavior and how it might impact his performance in school. His score on the Behavior Assessment System for Children (BASC) showed he was borderline ADHD. Also included in the packet was Matthew's report card.

"It looks like he's having some difficulty," I said.

Judy confirmed that he was struggling academically, which she suspected was due, at least in part, to the fact that he can't sit still. "If he's not up to sharpen his pencil, he's rummaging through his backpack. He'll return to his seat if asked, but in a few minutes, he's up again. And he's always talking—to a classmate, to himself, to someone passing in the hallway. If he thinks he knows the answer to a question, he just blurts it out."

After ruling out other causes for his fidgety behavior and impulsivity, Matthew fit the profile of a child with ADHD. But I wasn't convinced that medication alone would be the best step in treating him. While it's often effective, I find medication works best when paired with behavior modification.

Since his lack of focus and inability to sit still were having a serious impact on his schoolwork, I suggested that Judy talk further with his teacher and the school psychologist. Together, we could develop a program that would be geared specifically to the problems Matthew faced. The plan needed to include plenty of positive reinforcement, but with consistent consequences too—and strong follow-through at home so Matthew was always sure what was expected of him.

With any kind of reward system, it's important to discuss the ultimate goal and explain that it's about success, not failure, and rewards, not punishment. Using a chart provides a visible way of tracking progress. When a child sees that he has some control over his world, and receives positive reinforcement, his ability to succeed improves.

The basic plan for Matthew is one that can be helpful for many children. Just alter it to fit specific behavior problems and goals.

Matthew's Stay-Seated Game Plan (appropriate for ages 4–10)

- Start a gold-star chart at home. Ask Matthew to help design and create the chart.
- Explain that it will be used to help—not punish—behavior.
- Discuss the goals and how Matthew can reach them.
- Provide strategies to help Matthew self-regulate his impulse to fidget—raise his hand before speaking in class, request permission to leave his desk, take a front-row seat in class—so he focuses on the teacher, not other kids.
- Provide a stress ball to squeeze when he's feeling fidgety. It can help drain off enough energy so he can pay attention.
- Ask Matthew's teacher to provide a daily report, and add gold stars on the days he stays on-task at school.
- After five gold stars in a row, treat him to something he

really loves—a trip to his favorite pizza place, or to a baseball game.

Growing up with ADHD

If your child is diagnosed with ADHD, it's important to keep your perspective. While it is a chronic condition that will present some challenge throughout life, it's not a life sentence or barrier to future successes. The severity or frequency of overactive and impulsive behaviors could lessen over the long term.

The ADHD Medication Controversy

Are we overmedicating our kids? I think it's more important to ask: Have we found the drug that works best for a particular child? Medications have been shown to be a very effective way to treat this disorder. However, an advisory panel recently urged the FDA to place strong warnings on all stimulant drugs used to treat ADHD because of a potential risk of heart attacks, strokes, and sudden death in susceptible individuals.

Diagnosis and treatment of ADHD should take place only after an extensive evaluation of the child's academic, social, and emotional development by the physician. Be wary of any physician willing to prescribe medication without a thorough consultation.

Only then would I recommend using medication in addition to behavior modification.

Discuss all the options with your pediatrician or with a health-care practitioner trained in behavioral disorders. There are some alternative treatments for ADHD, including herbs, vitamins, chiropractic treatments, and optometric vision training. Although I know people who use them, I strongly urge caution since there's little evidence that they're effective, and some can be risky.

Finding the right treatment for a child with ADHD will make a tremendous difference each and every day—you'll see a happier, more self-confident child who is able to succeed in school and in life.

However, as a child becomes a teen and young adult, the need for medication usually continues.

Many children with ADHD become successful, creative adults who juggle multiple tasks with ease. Learning how to compensate for the disorder—by developing personal systems of organization, list making, time management, and stress reduction—helps children balance their internal lack of focus with the demands of the outside world. You can start instilling these habits early by doing a few things with your ADHD child as a team:

- Make sure he eats a well-rounded, healthy diet.
- Stick to a schedule that ensures enough sleep.
- Limit the distractions in his homework environment.
- Have him write down assignments and questions he has about them to ask you at home—to avoid repetitious questions in class. BUT assure him it's okay to ask some questions at school to be sure he understands instructions.
- Set up a graphic or visual organizer to help him keep track of assignments.

A Detour in Reading: Dyslexia

Children who have trouble learning to read may be struggling with dyslexia. There are other similar learning disabilities, by the way—dyscalculia, or difficulty with math concepts, and dysgraphia, or difficulty with writing. However, dyslexia is the most common cause of reading, spelling, and writing difficulties. It affects 5 to 10 percent of children in the United States, both girls and boys equally.

Dyslexia is a neurological problem that tends to run in families. So if other family members—parent, grandparents, aunts,

Early Warning Signs of Dyslexia

Catching learning disabilities like dyslexia early makes them easier to overcome. Here are some warning signs:

- Confusing left and right
- Difficulty pronouncing words
- Slow development of language
- Difficulty with rhyming and remembering words to songs
- Difficulty remembering sequences, such as the alphabet or months of the year
- Difficulty doing tasks in sequence
- Reading below grade level
- Difficulty reading aloud without making many errors
- Difficulty spelling, even when copying words (transposing letters is common)
- Confusing small words
- Difficulty following multistep directions
- Difficulty retelling stories

uncles—have dyslexia, pay particular attention to your child's reading development.

Environmental factors may play a role as well, but experts disagree on how much. Providing a language-rich environment can do a great deal to bolster literacy skills and facilitate the rapid cognitive development that occurs before age 3. But even the most attentive parents—those who read and speak to their children from infancy—can have a child with dyslexia. My conclusion? Genetics plays a larger role than the learning environment in determining whether a child will have dyslexia.

Early Identification Is Important

Children with dyslexia *can* learn to read, and with effective teaching beginning in kindergarten, they will be more likely to keep reading at their grade level through the years.

Children who aren't diagnosed and helped until the third grade often have more difficulty than kids who were identified earlier. It is common for them to still have trouble reading in the ninth grade. Clearly, the earlier dyslexia is caught, the better. But as usual, it's never too late (even for adults) to learn how to read. While there is no medical cure for dyslexia, with hard work and proper instruction, kids who have it can learn to compensate for the disorder, read well, and thrive academically and socially.

Raising a Lifelong Learner

Encouraging a love of learning is one of the greatest gifts you can give children. Although your level of involvement will change often—sometimes directing, sometimes stepping back—enriching their environment, ensuring needs are met, supporting them through challenging periods, and applauding every success are all essential to raising a lifelong learner.

As your children grow, share with them your enthusiasm for discovery:

- If you're excited about something you've read, discuss it over dinner.
- Embark on a new learning adventure together, perhaps tackling a new language. As you take a walk or run errands together, attempt to carry on a conversation in your second language.
- If something sparks your interest, jump in with both feet and involve your child. It might be figuring out your new digital camera or learning to play the piano.

Remember to instill a sense of perspective: Sometimes the best learning occurs when things don't come easily:

- If you're enrolled in an adult-ed class and are struggling to complete an assignment, let your child know how you plan to deal with it: Meet with the teacher? Do extra research? Spend some quiet time at the library? If your grade isn't what you'd hoped for, explain that you gave it your best effort and still learned something in the process.
- Ask kids to teach you something they already know how to do. Helping you learn—and seeing you stumble—gives them the opportunity to shine and lets you demonstrate patience and perseverance.

Seven Steps to Raising a Lifelong Learner

1. **Define their learning style.** Figure out if it's primarily:
   - Visual—learns best by seeing teacher demonstrations, diagrams on board, pictures in books.
   - Auditory—learns best by listening to lectures, discussions among classmates, even audio books.
   - Kinesthetic—learns best by doing, engaging with the environment, role playing.
2. **Enlist help.** Partner with your child's school to implement a program that encourages success.
3. **Keep focused.** Help your child work on what needs to be worked on first, finish it, and then move on.
4. **Celebrate success.** Praise kids often for what they're good at and encourage continued growth in those areas.
5. **Stay positive.** Don't allow children to define themselves by limitations: "I'm no good at math" or "I'm a bad reader."
6. **Track progress.** Spotlight how hard they try, how far they've come.
7. **Provide perspective.** Let them know that you make mistakes, that perfection isn't the goal, and that errors are an opportunity to learn.

- Celebrate learning. If you don't take perfect pictures with your new camera, who cares? You've captured some great memories. Laugh and enjoy them together, and promise you'll learn to do better.

All kids can become lifelong learners. Your unflagging encouragement and enthusiasm will make them want to open the door to the endless opportunities knowledge provides.

Intellectual Milestones:
What to Look for at Different Ages

Babyhood—7 to 12 Months

Ages 7 to 12 Months	Communication/ Language Skills	Cognitive/ Intellectual Skills
Babies at this age are curious about everything. As they become more coordinated, babies begin to interact more with the environment. Their memory improves, and they begin toying with independence—trying to feed themselves, for example. And those cute babbling sounds are actually the beginning of language development!	• Recognizes words for common items such as "cup," "shoe," and "juice" • Responds to name and to simple verbal cues such as "no" • Uses simple gestures such as shaking head for "yes" or "no" • Babbles with inflection, to imitate different speech sounds • Tries to communicate with actions or gestures • Says one or two words ("bye-bye," "dada," "mama," "no"), although they may not be clear • Uses exclamations such as "Oh-oh!"	• Explores objects in many different ways—for example, by shaking, banging, throwing, and dropping • Plays with two toys at once • Looks for dropped items—food on the floor, or a ball as it rolls away • Repeats an action that gets a reaction—for example, knocking over blocks • Finds a toy that is covered up • Enjoys looking at pictures in books • Enjoys games such as pat-a-cake and peek-a-boo

Toddlers—12 to 24 Months

Ages 12 to 24 Months	Communication/ Language Skills	Cognitive/ Intellectual Skills
This is a fun time for babies and parents alike. Not only are babies learning to walk, climb, and even dance, but they also are learning how to speak, respond to simple directions, and tell you what they want, usually by pointing. By the end of this stage, babies can use their fingers and hands to turn the pages of a book, stack blocks, and scribble with a crayon. They love repetitive songs and stories. Although they probably like to be around other kids, play is usually side by side rather than interactive. Learning to share comes later. Language skills are really developing at this stage, too—for example, linking two words together for simple sentences and using pronouns such as "me" and "mine."	• Listens to simple stories, songs, and rhymes • Follows simple commands and understands simple questions • Communicates likes and dislikes nonverbally or with simple language • Says several single words and repeats overheard words • Uses two-word sentences and questions—for example, "More juice," "Where kitty?" • Imitates new words and phrases such as "Go bye-bye," and "Mommy's car" • Sings songs in their own way • Points to items or body parts when named • Says some words that people outside the family can understand	• Understands how familiar objects are used, such as cups and spoons • Develops shape and size discrimination and starts sorting objects into similar groups • Shows excitement when completing simple tasks such as dropping blocks into a box • Realizes things exist when they are out of sight and can find objects even when hidden under two or three covers • Begins trying to help with activities such as feeding, undressing, and grooming • Begins wanting to hold books or turn pages • Begins solving simple problems • Recognizes him/herself and family in photos • Attempts simple two- or three-piece puzzles • Begins make-believe play such as feeding a doll or putting a teddy bear to sleep • Enjoys finger play, nonsense, and nursery rhymes

The Terrible Twos—2 to 3 Years

Ages 2 to 3	Communication/ Language Skills	Cognitive/ Intellectual Skills
The terrible twos? Perhaps children at this age developed a reputation for being terrible because they like to try to accomplish basic tasks independently, often refusing help. Kids at this age can be very stubborn and want to do things their own way, like getting dressed, eating, potty training, and washing hands. This is important for their development, and there's no harm in letting them try. Also, since kids can now speak in two- to four-word sentences, they can—and do!—express their feelings and frustrations.	• Follows two-part requests such as "Please get the book and bring it to me" • Understands differences in meaning such as "up-down" "go-stop," "big-little" • Has a word for almost everything • Uses simple two- to four-word sentences to talk about and ask for things • Often asks for or directs attention to objects by naming them • Can say name, age, and sex, and uses own name to refer to self • Uses pronouns such as "I," "you," "me," "we," "they," and some plurals • Uses plurals in a generalized way—for example, "foots" • Expresses feelings verbally • Is aware of how numbers sound and can count up to five • Uses size words correctly, such as "big" and "little" • Can be understood by most people outside the family	• Better understands similar and different shapes and sizes, and can sort groups of objects into sets • Participates in a wider range of activities such as exploring playground equipment, climbing on rocks, investigating cabinets, and thumbing through books • Can recognize and solve problems through active exploration, including trial and error • Can make mechanical toys work • Plays make-believe with dolls, animals, and people • Completes simple three- or four-piece puzzles

Preschoolers—3 to 4 Years

Ages 3 to 4	Communication/ Language Skills	Cognitive/ Intellectual Skills
Children at this age are much more aware of and confident about day-to-day activities. They enjoy structure and may be interested in going to preschool. Although they are learning how to play well with other children, they need guidance on taking turns and sharing. They can follow rules and are less likely to act on impulse. This is also a time for immense growth in language skills: Most 3-year-olds have over 700 words in their vocabulary!	• Correctly names some colors • Counts objects • Uses many sentences with four or more words • Tells simple stories • Whispers • Begins to master some basic rules of grammar • Understands position words such as "in," "out," and "behind" • Usually talks easily without repeating syllables or words • Asks many "what," "where," and "who" questions • Speaks clearly enough to be understood by people outside the family	• Classifies objects by purpose—for example, "to play with" or "to wear" • Recognizes and labels different shapes and matches simple geometric forms • Shows interest in a wider variety of tasks, activities, and experiences • Works to complete a task even if it is moderately difficult • Approaches problems from a single point of view • Engages in fantasy play • Understands concept of opposites • Understands time intervals better such as today, tomorrow, and yesterday • Can trace a square, copy a circle, and imitate horizontal strokes • Can put on own shoes, but not necessarily on the proper foot

The "Why?" Stage—4 to 5 Years

Ages 4 to 5	Communication/ Language Skills	Cognitive/ Intellectual Skills
If you're the parent of a 4-year-old, chances are you know how exhilarating and exasperating it can be. Not only are children at this age full of energy and the desire to test their physical limits, but they're also endlessly curious about the world around them. You probably hear "Why?" all day long.	• Can count ten or more objects • Can correctly name at least four colors • Communicates easily with other children and adults • Uses new and unfamiliar words • Understands complete sentences and forms sentences with more than one clause • Uses correct grammatical structure • Uses past, present, and future verbs such as "talked," "talk," and "will talk" • Uses negatives, for example, "I don't want to go to bed" • Tells longer stories and accurately relays information • Talks about imaginary people and occurrences • Plays with silly word combinations, recites rhymes, sings songs • Knows name and address • Starts to show interest in learning letters, shapes, and numbers • Asks "why" and "how" • Asks for word definitions • Says most speech sounds clearly and accurately except a few—typically l, s, r, v, z, j, ch, sh, th	• Begins understanding the difference between reality and fantasy and between something alive and an inanimate object • Understands how to sort and classify objects by characteristics and can begin matching pictures in simple games • Replicates patterns, sequences, and order • Understands concepts of nearest and farthest, more and less • Understands simple addition and subtraction • Understands the concept of time • Understands "parts," "whole," and "half" • Is increasingly able to focus attention, ignoring distractions and interruptions • Asks to participate in new experiences that he/she has seen or heard of • Is able to draw on varied resources when solving problems • Builds large, complex structures from blocks • Understands measurements such as weight, height, and length

Starting School—5 to 7 Years		
Ages 5 to 7	**Communication/ Language Skills**	**Cognitive/ Intellectual Skills**
The school-age years have begun. Now that kids are spending less time at home and more time at school, they are more and more influenced by teachers and peers. Not only is their intellectual growth becoming more complex, but they're beginning to operate in a bigger social realm. They're learning how to communicate with others and establish friendships, while developing moral reasoning and problem-solving skills outside of the classroom.	• Asks higher-level questions such as, "What would happen if . . . ?" • Sequences numbers • Uses increasingly complex descriptions • Engages in conversations that are more social and less egocentric • Uses a sentence length of approximately six words • Recites entire alphabet • Counts to one hundred by rote • Uses passive voice appropriately, such as "the last cookie was eaten by someone" • Is able to write upper- and lower-case letters • Writes expanding list of dictated letters and words	• Draws recognizable person, tree, and house, but pictures are not proportionate • Colors within lines • Understands "left" and "right" and clearly exhibits right- or left-handedness • Dresses independently • Can maintain focus on a project for a sustained period of time • Will return to an activity after being interrupted • Persists in completing longer-term or complex projects, with supervision • Uses self-motivation and other strategies to finish difficult tasks • Attempts wider range of new experiences, both independently and with peers and adults • May deliberately take risks when learning new skills • Is increasingly able to think of possible solutions to problems • Analyzes complex problems more accurately in order to identify the type of help needed

Elementary Learners—7 to 11 Years

Ages 7 to 11	Communication/ Language Skills	Cognitive/ Intellectual Skills
Learning happens quickly during this stage. Before you know it, kids in this age range will have mastered multiplication and long division, and be writing book reports and research papers. This is a great time for kids to learn accountability and responsibility when it comes to their work habits. Give them a planner to write down assignments and learn to manage time. These organizational skills will be of great benefit in the years ahead.	• Masters all speech sounds, including consonant blends • Appropriately controls rate, pitch, and volume of speech • Uses complex and compound sentences easily • Consistently uses correct grammar, including tense, pronouns, and plurals • Reads with considerable ease • Writes compositions • Is able to carry on complex conversations • Follows fairly complex directions with little need for repetition	• Has well-developed understanding of time and number concepts • Thinks about things in a more organized and logical manner • Is capable of concrete problem solving • Can think through actions and trace them back to events in order to explain situations • Can talk through problems in order to solve them • Can focus attention and take time to search for necessary information • Can develop a plan to meet a goal • Has increased memory capability

Tweens and Teens—11 to 18 Years

Ages 11 to 18	Communication/ Language Skills	Cognitive/ Intellectual Skills
Middle- and high-school-age kids are becoming independent learners and thinkers. At this age children often become passionate about subjects and interests that they can relate to. Whether they're enthusiastic about music, sports, literature, science, or history, encourage and support their interests and recognize that they're becoming the self-reliant, independent, and lifelong learners you've always hoped for.	• Comprehends and uses analogies and inductive and deductive reasoning • Understands metaphors and similes • Uses idioms and slang terms • Begins understanding ambiguity and sarcasm • Masters syntax • Continues to expand vocabulary • Seeks to interact with adults on a more mature level • Is increasingly able to engage in debate	• Initiates and carries out tasks without supervision • Begins to think in much broader terms, recognizing how things are connected to one another • Begins developing advanced reasoning skills, thinking through multiple options and possibilities • Begins developing abstract thinking skills, considering things that cannot be seen, heard, or touched • Begins examining internal feelings and thoughts • Sets goals based on personal needs and priorities • Explores topics of interest in depth • Enjoys playing with ideas • Demonstrates heightened level of self-consciousness • Can handle proportions, algebra, and other purely abstract processes • Begins seeking own solutions rather than asking adults for assistance

What Your Child's Teacher Needs to Know About Your Child

Your child is so much more than test scores and subject grades! In order to best teach your son or daughter, the teacher should know the following things:

☐ Child's name _____

☐ Child's birth date _____

☐ Is your child socially reserved or outgoing? _____

☐ Does your child have any special talents or interests? _____

☐ What is your child's learning style? More visual? Audio? Or does he or she learn best by doing?

_____

☐ Is your child easily distracted by others? Will he or she need to have a quiet spot to take
   tests, or a seat at the front of the class in order to work best?

_____

☐ Is your child an independent learner, or better in groups?

_____

☐ Has your child been diagnosed with anything that may affect academic performance—such
   as ADHD or dyslexia—or that may require frequent or extended absences?

_____

☐ What subjects is your child most interested in?

_____

☐ What subjects does your child need the most help with?

_____

☐ Are there any family/social situations that might affect your child's school performance,
   such as a separation or divorce, a new baby in the house, a history of being bullied?

_____

Things to Consider When Selecting a School for Your Child

School rankings are often based on the standardized test scores of the student body. While this is one good way to compare schools, don't select a school solely by numerical scores. Consider these three factors, too:	
Other Numbers	• What is the total enrollment? What is the teacher-to-student ratio? • Will your child get the special attention he or she needs? • What is the tuition? Are there scholarships available?
Special Programs	• Does the school have the resources to serve your child's specific academic needs, such as enrichment or special ed programs, resource rooms, or after-school tutoring? • Does the school offer art programs? Music? Drama? • Does the school have a physical education program? • How healthy and well-balanced is the lunch program? • Does the school have an active parent–teacher organization?
Practical Matters	• Are there other enrollment requirements, such as an interview process? • Does the school provide transportation? Is the location convenient? • How safe and secure is the school?

Many of the charts and checklists in this chapter can be printed out at
www.RealAge.com/parenting

Chapter 6

CHIN UP
Routines That Build Up Your Child's Self-Esteem
("accentuate the positive, eliminate the negative" is still good advice)

You've probably noticed that kids' interests, abilities, and personalities are as unique as their looks. For example, while one child is quiet and spends every spare moment curled up with a book, another loves having an audience and telling stories, and yet another is always taking things apart and putting them back together again.

But do you know what all three kids have in common?

By exploring their interests and honing their strengths, each one is building self-esteem and self-image—their inner sense of self. Emotional health is as important as physical health. A child's well-being includes a healthy body *and* a healthy mind—and when there is trouble in one area, the other is affected. Parents lay the groundwork upon which kids build self-confidence, self-control, self-worth, and self-esteem.

A positive sense of self will help your child cope with stressful situations, from peer pressure to moving to a new town.

Let's step back and figure out how healthy your child's self-esteem is before we get into the nitty-gritty. In the Real-Age Healthy Kids Test, you were asked, "**How do you think your child would rate his/her overall self-worth or self-image?**" This can be a difficult question to answer if your child is under 8, as these traits are still far from formed. To help evaluate whether your answer was right on, consider a few more questions:

1. How does my child feel about his/her overall appearance?
    a. Attractive most of the time
    b. Attractive some of the time
    c. Average
    d. Not so attractive
    e. Unattractive
    f. Not sure

2. How athletic does my child consider himself/herself to be?
    a. Outstanding
    b. Above average
    c. Average
    d. Below average
    e. Not at all athletic
    f. Not sure

3. Does my child feel accepted by his/her peers?
    a. Yes, absolutely
    b. Yes, mostly
    c. Sometimes
    d. Not usually
    e. Never
    f. Not sure

4. How would my child describe his/her performance in school?

    a. Excellent

    b. Above average

    c. Average

    d. Below average

    e. Not at all scholastic

    f. Not sure

5. How does my child view his/her behavior?

    a. Perfect kid

    b. Really good kid

    c. Pretty good kid

    d. Gets in trouble sometimes

    e. Troublemaker

    f. Not sure

Researchers have shown that these five questions help reveal how children judge themselves and compare themselves with others. The answers give you a good idea of your child's overall sense of self-worth.

If any of your answers were "not sure," go on a mission to find out. You'll have to do some detective work and read between the lines, but the understanding you'll gain will be worth it.

What Is Good Self-Esteem, Anyway?

Some self-doubt is healthy. It enhances your child's safety.

It starts with a balanced, realistic sense of who you are and what you are capable of. Having this helps kids find their niche—the place where they feel like they belong and have something to contribute. A bit of self-doubt is important. Kids shouldn't think they're invincible. This can be quite dangerous, especially in teens celebrating their first driver's license. Realizing that there are boundaries can help keep them from getting injured.

At the same time, you don't want your children to be afraid of what life has to offer. They need to challenge themselves, work hard, and be the best they can be. You can help by guiding them toward activities that play to their strengths and offer them opportunities to shine. Kids develop good, healthy self-esteem by mastering different skills and gaining more control over their environment, not by simply being told that they're good at something or that they're attractive or smart.

In fact, one tricky aspect of building a child's self-esteem is that you can't give empty praise. Children are adept at detecting little white lies, and if they hear them they will start to disbelieve other things you say. So be honest. When you see your child doing something good, be quick with praise.

> Eliminate empty praise . . . your kids will be on to you in a flash.

On the other hand, keep your antennae up. If an average-looking child asks if she's beautiful, an answer like, "You're beautiful on the inside, honey," will be heard as "You're an ugly duckling." An honest and heartfelt "I think you're *more* than beautiful" can work wonders for a child who's unsure about her features.

Here's something else to keep in mind: The ultimate goal is to give your child a sense of self-worth that doesn't need constant praise or rewards. It's fine to stick gold stars on charts when young children do all their chores or floss every day. But as kids get older, they should start to develop a sense of pride in doing what's expected and doing it well.

The Price for Low Self-Esteem

Although it's hard to measure low self-esteem in a scientific sense, studies show that it can be a risk factor for suicide,

What do the answers say about your child's self-esteem?

Mostly a's: If your child is under age 7 or 8, you probably answered mostly a's and/or e's. That's because younger children see things as either good or bad, and don't compare themselves with others. Instead, they compare what they used to be able to do to what they can do now: "I didn't know how to ride a bike last year, but now I can!" As a result, young children's views of themselves tend to be very favorable, which is great.

A child over 8 for whom you answered mostly a's has strong self-esteem. Just be sure that she also views the world realistically and doesn't think she's invincible, so she doesn't endanger her safety.

Mostly b's: Most kids under 12 fall into this category, although some teens do as well. A child who feels she's a pretty good kid realizes that there may be others who are smarter, prettier, and more athletic, but she still maintains a high self-worth. However, some kids over 12 start to question their value.

Mostly c's: A kid who believes, rightly or wrongly, that he is both good and bad might be struggling to control his life. Does he feel he can change if he wants to? Does he beat himself up without cause? Finding out why a child feels split and torn can help you determine what is needed to boost his ego.

Mostly d's: Children who get mostly d's are sliding into a cycle of negative self-esteem. It could be a phase or the start of a pattern. Once children hit their tweens and teens, they begin to recognize their limitations as well as their strengths. This is when self-image can slide. They may not feel they measure up academically or socially. If they see themselves as outside of the "popular group" they may try too hard to fit in, or blow perceived flaws out of proportion.

It's important to improve their sense of worth. This chapter can get you started, but if you don't see a difference within a few weeks, ask your pediatrician to recommend a therapist who specializes in children.

Mostly e's: A child with a negative self-image who doesn't respond to anything you say or do can be heading for serious trouble. Plunging self-esteem has been linked to depression, eating disorders, behavioral problems, and suicide. Don't take a wait-and-see attitude; get professional help. Too many kids try to hurt themselves . . . and some succeed. Some talk therapy can get to the bottom of your child's problems and provide strategies for the whole family to help. There's more insight later in this chapter, too.

depression, teenage pregnancy, and eating disorders in kids as young as 10 or 11. While it may not be the only factor, it's one you can strongly influence. For example, researchers have found that a number of things can contribute to a depressive episode during adolescence, including:

- Low self-esteem
- Physical, psychological, and social changes that accompany this age and stage
- A significant transition, change, or loss (moving, divorce of parents, death)

You can't stop your kids from going through puberty, and you may not always have control over changes in your family structure, but you *can* help boost their self-esteem.

Stages for a Healthy Development of Self

The development of a healthy sense of self is a complex process that begins in babies and continues into early adulthood and beyond. While the process varies from child to child, there are general milestones in each age group that parents can greatly influence by being consistent, nurturing, and responsive . . . even when your kids insist they don't need you anymore! (You can skip ahead to the age group that applies to your child: baby, toddler, young child, older child, tween, and teen.)

Babies (under 2)

In the first year of life, babies begin to realize they are individuals, and start to distinguish themselves from others. They realize they have a certain amount of control over their world and recognize cause and effect. A baby who drops a toy from the high chair learns that someone will pick it up again and *again*. This can become a baby's favorite game!

Loving interactions with your child now will lay the groundwork for a positive self-image later. But infants who lack a secure bond with the people who care for them may be more prone to a negative self-image in the years ahead, and possibly depression.

Toddlers (2–4)

A big milestone for toddlers is recognizing themselves in mirrors and pictures. At around 2, they begin to express themselves verbally and behave independently, making separation easier. They also develop some sense of self-control—though they don't always use it!

As they work toward more independence, toddlers test boundaries, learning what they can and cannot do. While it's easy to become frustrated when they yell "No!" for the 1,273rd time, toddlers aren't just trying to be difficult. They're asserting themselves, which is actually an important and healthy stage in the development of self. Try dealing with these power struggles by offering kids a couple of choices: "Would you like to wear the red shirt or the blue one?" "Should we go to the park or the beach today?" This gives children some sense of autonomy without letting them run the show.

Early Childhood (5–8)

Kids this age start rating themselves in five areas: physical ability, appearance, acceptance by peers, mental ability, and overall behavior. They are very black-and-white about it. They are either "good" or "bad" athletes, "good" or "bad" readers. They don't recognize that there are gray areas or that their abilities may vary with the situation.

Although kids do acknowledge similarities and differences among their peers, their greatest measure of achievement is not comparing their achievements with others, but comparing what they can do now with what they could do when they were younger.

Kids at this age tend to have a very high, perhaps even unrealistic, perception of themselves, so low self-esteem is rarely an issue. But eventually they finally start to gain a little perspective—things are not always all or nothing. They'll start saying things like, "I am somewhat good at making friends," or "I'm okay at taking tests."

Middle Childhood (8–12)

Children at this age begin to have broader, more balanced views of themselves and are able to see both their limitations and strengths. This can be a blessing and a curse, as they begin to compare themselves with others and be more self-critical. They may be uneasy about how competent they are at school, question their value as a family or community member, or wonder if they have what it takes to succeed in life. Watch out for too many negative feelings around now.

How they feel about themselves also depends on their ability to make friends. Social acceptance plays a major role in developing and maintaining self-esteem, and friendships start to assume a pivotal role now. They provide a wide range of development opportunities for children, including group problem solving and managing conflicts.

Early to Middle Adolescence (13–15)

Around this age, kids start to evaluate themselves psychologi-cally—they begin to have complex views about their emo-

How Teenagers Define Themselves

One of the most important psychological developments in teens is forming a sense of identity. Coming to understand who they are and how they fit into this world is no easy task. A recent study found that teens use their past life—their memories so far, good or bad—to make sense of where they are and where they're headed. A life that's been filled with meaningful, positive experiences helps kids form a positive sense of identity.

tions and beliefs, and to think in abstract terms. Self-esteem generally increases at this age—but so do mood swings. Whether these emotional roller coasters are due to changing hormones or the struggle to understand themselves (or, more likely, both), they're a normal part of self-development.

But pay close attention if moodiness becomes dark and extreme. Adolescents who feel chronically pessimistic may be clinically depressed and need psychological help. Sound too close for comfort? Skip ahead to the section in this chapter on depression to learn more.

Late Adolescence (16–18)

All of those emotional ups and downs are finally beginning to resolve. Kids have a more balanced, accurate view of themselves and are well on their way to establishing their self-identity. They have more self-esteem than younger children, who have yet to reach the same level of self-awareness, and they're confident about sharing that identity with others.

Five Ways to Give Your Child an Emotional Boost

You may be thinking, "My child has great self-esteem. She's found activities she enjoys and excels in. She's doing well in school and has plenty of friends. No problems here." That's wonderful. But it may not last. Many children go through patches of self-doubt that can last for a week, a couple of months, or spiral into years. If things start going wrong, here are some ways to try to help set them right, quickly.

1. **Encourage your child to get physical.**

   Studies show that exercise has at least a short-term positive effect on self-esteem in children. For instance, when researchers compared more than 1,800 children ages 3 to 20, those who began exercising had more self-esteem in just four weeks. Try to find an activity that interests your child, then be ready with transportation, encouragement, equipment—whatever it takes. This will involve effort, time, and expense, but the benefits can be tremendous. (See Chapter 3 for tips on exercise motivation.)

> **Write It Down**
>
> While parents would love it if our kids always came to us when they're having a problem, this isn't realistic—especially with older kids who are fighting to establish their independence.
>
> One way to help them sort through confusing feelings on their own is to encourage kids—even those as young as 7—to keep a daily journal or diary. Often just putting their thoughts down on paper helps them find insights and gain perspective. It works for adults too, by the way. . . .

2. **Get help at school.**

   If academics seem to be part of the problem, check with the school for recommendations. Some schools have homework helpers to work with kids who need extra teaching time. If yours doesn't, ask for tutoring recommendations—there may be a qualified college student or retired teacher in the neighborhood who does tutoring and can help get your child back on track with the rest of the class.

3. **Nurture healthy habits.**

   Low self-esteem can sometimes be caused by kids getting into a cycle of not taking care of themselves, and busy parents thinking it's just a weird phase—until it becomes more than that. Nip these patterns in the bud. Enforce bedtimes with younger kids and make sure older ones get enough ZZZZs to function properly. Ditto for regular showers and shampoos— iffy personal hygiene can turn off other kids, socially isolating anyone who's "gross." Check what they're eating with an eye toward imbalances, or getting energy spikes—and then crashes—from caffeinated sodas and sweets. At home, insist on eating fresh, healthy meals together (see Chapter 2).

4. Reward accomplishments.
Emphasize the positive. Play up a good test score or a completed essay; hand out stars for a successful piano lesson. If your child is discouraged in one area, such as sports or math, make a big deal of accomplishments in another, such as reading or drawing.

5. Do something just for fun.
Surprise your child by planning a breakfast cookout, a trip to an amusement park, an evening at the movies, or even a weekend getaway to an air and space museum. Especially if something like peer pressure is getting him down, doing something that's out of the blue and all about him will make him feel special and give him something to tell the world about.

Dig a Little Further

Now that we've gone over one of the test's key concerns—overall self-worth—let's look at your answers to the rest of the emotional health questions.

Which family activities do you and your child enjoy frequently?
You are your children's biggest role model. Your principles and

beliefs shape how they view themselves. So *any* time you spend with them is a positive thing: walking, shopping, playing ball, using the video-cam, even doing chores together (although this may not be your kid's *favorite* thing to do with you)—it doesn't really matter what it is.

True Parenting Story:
Finding One-on-One Time with Two Kids

Amy, my daughter, loves to do things with me and she often asks if we can take a bike ride, go out for ice cream, or catch a movie. That's wonderful, but not long ago I realized that my son, Scott, gets far less one-on-one time with me—he tends to hang back a little, and when he does suggest doing something together, my daughter often tags along.

Then a few weeks ago Scott spotted some local ads for garage sales that mentioned baseball cards. He collects them and asked if we could hit some sales together. Amy laughed and said no way was she getting up early on a weekend to look at someone else's junk. So Scott and I drove around all Saturday morning, found two cards he'd been wanting, and ended up at the bagel store where we had a great one-on-one talk. Now we're planning to make this a regular thing.

Scott is talking to me more in general as a result. I think he just needed to feel that he's as important to me as his sister is. Who knew garage sales would make that happen?

CHELSEA, RYE BROOK, NY

How often does your child come to you for help with a problem?

Often, I hope. Not that you should be your child's best friend. But you should be available to listen, ask questions, and advise any time. This can sometimes be tricky, especially as adolescents become autonomous and even secretive. Just let your kids know that you are there whenever for whatever and, fingers crossed, they'll come to you with their troubles.

But besides being approachable, you need to provide boundaries. Parents who are affectionate, involved, and encouraging but who also set and enforce clear rules tend to have children with higher self-worth than children with superstrict, controlling parents.

That said, it's pretty much a given that eventually there will be some things your children absolutely won't talk to you about—but they might talk to another adult. You'll be ahead of the game if you indirectly suggest a confidante or two, maybe an admired teacher or a hip godparent.

How many extended family members does your child maintain contact with (through visits, e-mail, phone calls, etc.)? Whether your extended family lives two miles away or 2,000 miles away, cell phones, computers, and fax machines make it unbelievably easy to stay in touch—and feeling the unconditional love family members offer is wonderful for a child's developing sense of self.

Help your children nurture those family bonds by having them write Grandma and Grandpa e-mails or send artwork over the fax machine. Put cousins, aunts, and uncles on speed dial so children can call at the touch of a button. Or form a family Internet group such as those offered on Yahoo! and then have fun posting notes and sharing photos. Not only will your children benefit from staying connected, your family will love it, too.

RealAge Projection: **Kids who have close connections with parents, grandparents, siblings, and other relatives generally struggle less with depression and peer pressure. And when** they become adults, these bonds can help them look and feel almost 4 years younger. Imagine that: your child, 40 years old, but feeling 36.

Getting Your Kids to Really Listen!

1. **Say your child's name first.** It gets their attention. "Sophia, please get ready for bed," is more effective than "Please get ready for bed, Sophia."

2. **Get within arm's length.** Don't holler to your child from across the house (or even across a room) and expect the message to get through. Instead, get close enough for your child to see your face clearly and focus on you instead of a roomful of distractions.

3. **Turn negatives into positives.** Kids hear "No" and "Don't" all day and begin to tune out the negative. Make those instructions positive and tell your child what to *do:* "Do hang up your coat," not "Don't drop your coat on the floor" or "Do finish your homework now," not "Don't touch the TV until your homework is done."

4. **Recognize your child's limits.** Most kids have trouble remembering more than three things at a time. Rather than giving them a laundry list of things to do, stop at three.

5. **Be courteous.** Speak to your child in the same way you would like to be spoken to. If you model good behavior, including using the "magic" words— *please, thank you,* and *you're welcome*—your child will learn to speak courteously and respectfully.

6. **Be consistent.** Being clear about rules will help your child meet your expectations. Waffling—allowing your son to ride his bike without a helmet one day and then insisting he wear it the next, for example—causes confusion.

7. **Give them a minute.** Children's brains take a bit of extra time to process information, so allow what you've said to sink in for a moment before you expect kids to get in gear.

8. **Be a good listener.** Model good listening habits whenever your child talks to you so you and others get the same treatment back. Good communication is a two-way street.

How well does your child play with siblings and children in the same age group?

One thing's sure: When it comes to self-esteem, friendships matter. It isn't important whether your child has two dozen friends or one treasured best friend. One is all it takes to boost a child's self-esteem, to feel worthwhile.

That's why it's crucial that kids develop the social skills—from starting conversations to solving conflicts—that will help them make and maintain friendships throughout their life. Teach kids how important it is to be kind, trustworthy, and loyal to friends, even at the youngest ages.

Making New Friends

Some kids have a knack for attracting and keeping friends. But others are on the shy side and may need a little help meeting potential pals and then breaking the ice. Here's where you come in:

- **Come up with conversation starters.** If your child wants to get to know a certain schoolmate but doesn't know how to go about it, suggest things the two could work on in common—a tricky math assignment or class art project.
- **Find meeting places.** Look for local activities your child may enjoy, such as a firehouse cookout or a street fair. Go with your child and introduce yourself—and her—to other families there.
- **Volunteer together.** If your kid is an animal lover, check out opportunities to help out at the local shelter; your child may make a new friend while filling water dishes. Over the holidays, stock shelves at the neighborhood food pantry.

- **Make a date.** To turn acquaintances into friends, suggest a pizza dinner and videos at your home. You can call the parents first to work out a time, then your child can e-mail or phone the friend-to-be.

Choosing Friends

Help your child recognize the qualities that make a good friend. Ask . . .

- What's your friend like?
- What do you like best about him?
- Does he treat people nicely?
- Is he loyal to you always or just sometimes?
- Is he generous? How? Or why not?
- Does he tell the truth?

How well do you think your child deals with peer pressure? What parent wouldn't want children who paddled against the stream and instinctively stood up for themselves? But it's not that easy. Peer pressure is a natural, and powerful, part of childhood that can begin as early as kindergarten.

Sometimes, of course, peer pressure is a good thing. Your child may join a sports team or school club or study group because "everyone's doing it."

But the negative side of peer pressure is no fun.

Kids want to feel liked and part of the crowd. (Don't we all?) If *all* the kids are wearing sparkly purple sneakers, your child will probably beg for a pair, too. Although this type of peer influence may seem harmless, the earlier you teach kids to make up their own mind, the easier it will be later for them to hold firm on things that really matter—especially saying "no" to smoking, drinking, and drugs.

A healthy self-esteem and the ability to cope with peer pressure go hand in hand. Kids who believe that their opinion is worthwhile will have an easier time asserting it.

Encourage children to think for themselves by bringing up a few hypothetical questions. Make it casual . . . maybe while you're walking the dog or washing the car together. Then ask:

- What would you do if you saw a classmate being bullied?
- What would you do if you realized a classmate was copying your answers on a math test?
- What would you do if some kids formed a club during recess and invited you to join, but not your best friend?

Then talk about each situation and brainstorm possible solutions together.

As your children enter adolescence, start to prepare them for the onslaught of peer pressure that usually comes with it by working on these two issues:

1. **Saying no.** Role-play how to turn down cigarettes, drugs, and alcohol. Kids who have practiced saying "no" are more likely to be able to say "no" when the real situation occurs.

2. **Choosing healthy friendships.** Remind your children that positive peer pressure can overcome negative. Kids who hang out with a group of friends who are a good influence are less tempted to spend time with kids who could be a bad influence.

If you talk about standing up to peer pressure early and often, when the tough decisions come—and they will—your kids are much more likely to make the right choice.

True Parenting Story:
When Other Kids Put the Pressure On

When my daughter Alice was in the second grade, she began to have a rough time on the playground. She wanted to play with a particular group of girls, but they'd include her one day and then exclude her the next, seemingly on a whim. One day, when she'd been rejected again, Alice's second-grade teacher, Ms. Baker, phoned to tell me that Alice was in tears, sobbing because the girls said they didn't want to be her friend.

I knew that I couldn't protect Alice from every ounce of hurt she would have growing up. But I could help to nurture her self-esteem so that when a cruel situation arose again, she wouldn't feel as helpless as she did that day.

That night, after a long talk with many tears and countless hugs, I gave Alice an assignment. "Tomorrow at recess," I began, "ask someone you've never played with before if she'd like to play with you. Then, when you come home from school, I want to hear all about it."

Alice bounded off the school bus the following afternoon with a huge grin. "I did it!" she exclaimed proudly. "I asked Kimberly if she wanted to play with me and we picked wildflowers for Ms. Baker during recess. She said they were beautiful."

This wasn't the last playground struggle for Alice, but from then on things seemed to change for her. I continue to remind Alice what it means to be a good friend, and how often being kind to others not only makes them feel good, but also makes you feel good.

—DIANE, BROOKLYN, NY

Is It Low Self-Esteem or Is It Depression?

How do you tell the difference between moody "growing pains" and depression? Time is one sign: Being sad or angry for an hour or two, or even a day or two, is pretty normal. Feeling sad for weeks or months is not. Another sign is not being able to function normally in day-to-day activities. Also, if there's a history of depression in your family, take any signs—including the ones below—even more seriously:

- Irritability and loss of temper over small things
- Recklessness
- Destruction of household items or toys
- Frequent outbursts of complaining or shouting
- Statements such as, "I hate myself"
- Chronic boredom or restlessness
- Persistent problems concentrating or constant daydreaming
- Loss of interest in previously enjoyed activities
- Hypersensitivity to failure and rejection
- Self-injury by biting, hitting, or cutting
- Changes in sleep patterns
- Changes in eating patterns
- Talk about death and suicide; statements such as, "I wish I were dead"

If your child is exhibiting any of these signs, seek professional help. **If your child is talking about suicide, get help** *immediately*. **Treat this as an emergency.**

A child psychiatrist may recommend therapy and often medication as well to treat depression. Follow treatment plans faithfully. Rarely, if ever, will a professional recommend drugs without therapy. Make sure your child takes the prescribed medications every day, despite assertions of "I feel fine." Be aware that having one bout of depression makes another one more likely. Episodes of depression often come and go in periods throughout a person's life. Without treatment, the risks can be extremely serious.

If your child develops depression, learn all you can about this condition. Join support groups and network with other parents going through the same experience. A depressed child may shut you out, but don't take it personally. Make it clear that you are available to listen *anytime* your child wants to talk. This is a message that you may need to convey over and over because a depressed child probably feels unworthy of love and attention. Meanwhile, provide a structured environment by sticking to daily routines, mealtimes and bedtimes. Be firm and consistent.

Overall, how confident is your child?

It's normal for children's confidence to ebb and flow as they grow up. Childhood is a time of many transitions, and even very confident children have periods of self-doubt. The shifts from elementary school to middle school, and from middle school to high school, can be especially anxious.

For example, a 12-year-old who once ruled the sixth grade is suddenly the youngest kid in a brand-new school, and is dealing with new expectations, academically and socially. Try reminding kids who get a little freaked how short the school year is in comparison with their whole life and, sooner than they think, it will all change.

As kids grow older, their confidence grows as well, in part because they gain more autonomy at school—choosing classes based on their interests and abilities, making independent friendships, steadily exploring and forming their own identity. Even if younger kids lack confidence, chances are good that will change. For now, encourage and praise their strengths.

How often does your child try new activities?

The more things kids try, the more likely they are to find an activity they love and excel at. Trying new things also gives children's confidence a boost, even if a particular activity doesn't turn into a passion.

Don't force kids to stick with something they discover they don't particularly enjoy. If you've paid for six weeks of gymnastics classes, there's no harm in having your child finish the session—who knows, she might change her mind halfway through. But if gymnastics truly turns out not to be her thing, try something else. Guitar lessons? Track and field? Just be sure your child understands this is all about experimentation and exploration, not failure. Talk about how we all learn from experience and make light of it, saying, for example, "Well! Now we can rule out speed skating as your life's pursuit!" A closed door on one activity can open a new door on something more exciting. Check out the local rec center's classes for new things to try—there's always something.

The Big Stresses—Self Esteem Will Help Get Them Through

Kids who have a strong sense of self-esteem are not only more likely to cope well with the little pressures—a new babysitter, homework deadlines—but with the biggies such as death, trauma, or divorce. They're less likely to blame themselves, or feel completely lost and abandoned. And they'll bounce back faster.

Still, most kids need some help getting through really difficult times, even those with Superman self-esteem. When life gets rough, identifying whether your child has too much stress to handle alone should be a priority. The box on page 197 includes eighteen of the biggest stressors kids can face. If your child is dealing with more than a few of them, some extra help and guidance from you—and possibly from a professional counselor—will help him get through it in good shape.

The lower your child's stress levels, the healthier your child will be—physically and emotionally. Stress not only can cause psychological difficulties, but it may also manifest itself in physical symptoms, including headaches, stomachaches, difficulty breathing, and a weakened immune system.

Children deal with stress in different ways, depending on their age, development, and mind/body state—for instance, a child who is tired may react in a different manner from a rested one, and vice versa. But some children are just more sensitive to stress than others. While one kid may shrug off a bad day at school, another may spend hours worrying about going back the next day. How your child handles tense situations may be just a part of his or her makeup, possibly inherited from family traits.

Eighteen Common Childhood Stressors

Divorce or separation of parents
Schoolwork/homework problems
Low grades
Disagreements with parents
Peer pressure: alcohol, cigarettes, drugs, sex
New stepfamily members introduced into home
Loss of pet
Change in day care
Move to a different home
Move to a different town
Move to a different school
New baby in home
Loss of family member or close friend
Rejection from team or club
New driver's license
Violence in school or neighborhood
Rejection by close friends
Health issues (the child's or a significant person's)

Helping Kids Tame Tension

Fears in childhood are normal. Be an attentive, patient listener and allow your children to talk about what frightens them. Discussing an upcoming event well ahead of time—like a visit to the doctor's office, for example—will help kids mentally prepare for it. Try reading a children's book together about what a doctor's checkup entails, or even play pretend about what's likely to happen. Often, what children fear the most is the unknown; eliminating the mystery can minimize the anxiety.

Changes in routine can also frazzle some kids, who like familiar and predictable environments, whereas others love spontaneity and change. When scheduling family life, try to find a happy medium. It may be tempting to rush from school to soccer to play rehearsal to homework to bedtime, but that kind of daily schedule will stress out any child. Plan for downtimes when kids can play quietly in their bedroom, read, do a craft project, or just "veg."

When Bad Things Happen

The concept of remaining calm for the children's sake is a good one in a bad situation. Studies have shown that in traumatic circumstances, such as wars or earthquakes, children tend to cope as well or as poorly as their parents do. A parent who falls apart may trigger even more fears in their children. But if you can keep it together, your kids will feel more secure and will even learn something about how to remain in control during difficult times.

> Parents who overreact in a stressful situation may spark irrational fears in their children.

Children need love and affection more than ever during and after traumatic incidents. They may suffer from depression, post-traumatic stress disorder, sleep problems, irrational fears, thinking that the incident will happen again, regressive behavior, excessive attachment to parents, and more. Professional help is often a must.

True Parenting Story:
When Trauma Strikes Close to Home

A few years ago, our home was burglarized while we were out for the day. My son Stevie was 9 at the time. Two of the things the thieves took were his most prized possessions: his PlayStation video game system and a baseball with autographs all over it. In the process, they made a mess of his room.

Based on what was stolen, the robbers were probably teenagers—they rummaged through the kids' closets, took toys of little value, and helped themselves to sodas and snacks.

I was angry, but I wasn't really worried that they would return. Stevie, on the other hand, began to obsess over it. For weeks afterward, each time we left the house he would double- and triple-check the locks. At night, he would be frightened by any unusual sound. I talked to Stevie's pediatrician, and he reassured me that my son's reaction was normal and would ease over time, but he also suggested taking him to a counselor, to see if talking it out might resolve his feelings more quickly.

The therapy sessions really helped make Stevie feel safer in our home. We also installed a home security system, which helped everyone's peace of mind. Soon afterward, I felt like my son was back to his old spirited self, researching the latest video game systems and plotting out which autographs to get on a new baseball.

—CHRISTINE, BRONXVILLE, NY

When Is Professional Help Needed?

How can you judge whether your child is stressed to the point of needing expert help? The chart on the next page lays out some practical guidelines.

How Children React to Stress at Different Ages

Age	Possible Reactions to Stress	When to Consider Professional Help
Toddler and Preschool (Ages 1–5)	• Increased attachment to parents • Frantic when left alone • Excessive crying • Shows regressive behavior (e.g., tantrums, sleeping problems) • Irritability • Eating problems • Confusion • Sensitivity to environment, especially noise • Quavering with fear	• Any reactions to stress that are prolonged or severe • No improvements despite extra care from parent/caregiver • Unusually quiet, detached
Early to Middle Childhood (Ages 5–11)	• Has difficulty sleeping • Has academic problems • Develops unreasonable fears • Has frequent gastrointestinal upsets, headaches/migraines • Shows regressive behavior (e.g., bed wetting, thumb sucking) • Avoids social interaction • Seems distracted, unfocused • Is irritable, combative • Is withdrawn	• Any reactions to stress that are prolonged or severe • Repeated bed-wetting • Overly anxious, unable to relax • Unable to leave parent(s) • Bouts of crying unrelated to any event
Early Adolescence (Ages 11–14)	• Seems withdrawn • Avoids interactions with family, friends • Has frequent gastrointestinal upsets, headaches/migraines, unexplainable aches and pains	• Any reactions to stress that are prolonged or severe • Profound depression— continually sad, despairing • Preoccupation with death, talks about suicide • Defiance, acting out, frequently aggressive • Refusal or inability to take care of basic needs: eating, drinking, bathing • Abuse of drugs, alcohol

Age	Possible Reactions to Stress	When to Consider Professional Help
Adolescence (Ages 14–18)	• Is withdrawn • Avoids interactions with family, friends • Has difficulty focusing on tasks • Has nightmares, or sleeps excessively • Responds physicallly (e.g., skin irritations, gastrointestinal upsets, headaches)	• Any reactions to stress that are prolonged or severe • Profound depression— continually sad, despairing • Refusal or inability to take care of basic needs: eating, drinking, bathing • Abuse of drugs, alcohol • Indecision • Obsessive behavior/thoughts • Hallucinations • Talk of suicide, harming others • Antisocial behavior (e.g., shoplifting, fighting)

If you decide your child needs help, ask your pediatrician or family doctor to recommend a professional who specializes in kids your child's age and has a child psychology background. Your child's school or other parents are also often good sources for recommendations.

Strong Emotional Health Through the Years

The self-esteem and coping mechanisms children develop in childhood will stick with them throughout the often tumultuous teen years and into adulthood. They will help them succeed in making good friends, achieving a rewarding career, and creating a healthy family of their own one day.

But as with physical health, don't take emotional wellness for granted. Children's outlook on life and sense of self can change from day to day as well as year to year; they may need firm guidance one week, and lots of extra cuddles and attention the next. Just remember that while they all have their down days, your overall goal is to infuse your kids with a positive, healthy, optimistic approach to life. That's success for them and for you as a parent.

Many of the charts and checklists in this chapter can be printed out at
www.RealAge.com/parenting

Chapter 7

GEAR UP
Habits That Keep Kids from Getting Hurt
(including the number one piece of protective sports gear)

Your 7-year-old rockets up a flight of hardwood stairs in his socks while carrying a stack of folded laundry—and suddenly you hear, "Ouch!" He crashes down on his knees on the fourth step with all the force of a semitruck.

You come running. "Oh, if only he weren't always in such a hurry, or hadn't kicked off his sneakers, this wouldn't have happened," you think, and you're probably right.

How annoying. You know it was avoidable, and you could've done something to stop it. Like installing those nonslip tread strips you saw at Home Depot or simply reminding him to put on his shoes and take his time. Somehow knowing that the incident was avoidable makes you feel even worse about those big bruises on his knees.

> Accidental injuries are the most common cause of death in children between ages 1 and 14.

The truth is that most accidents aren't accidents at all. They don't happen by chance; they happen because we overlook, underestimate, or ignore risky situations.

In a word, we get careless.

Now all kids have plenty of opportunities to find trouble. And they do. The statistics are overwhelming: Accidental injuries are by far the most common cause of death in children ages 1 to 14, taking more lives than birth defects, cancers, violence, and heart disease combined. In addition, accidents leave thousands of kids permanently disabled or disfigured each year.

These statistics are scary, but the last thing to do is overreact and swear to never let your kids out of your sight. Studies show that most childhood injuries can be avoided by consistently following basic precautions and taking simple steps (so to speak) to make their surroundings safe. Clearly, it isn't possible to prevent absolutely every injury, but it is possible to bring the risks way down.

When Do Most Accidents Happen?

Good bet you think during the school day, when kids are out of the house and away from your vigilant eyes. Wrong.

Most childhood accidents occur in the late afternoon and early evening, on weekends, during the summer, and on school holidays.

Home Safe Home

Begin by making sure your home is as safe as possible. You probably completely baby-proofed it before your first child arrived, but as kids grow older and families expand, we tend to forget how important home safety is.

In fact, after taking the online RealAge Healthy Kids Test at www.RealAge.com/parenting, one mom commented: "This online test reminded me of the importance of safety in the home, not just of having physically healthy kids. With my firstborn, I was super aware of child-proofing issues, but now, with three little ones, I have gotten kind of relaxed. We are getting new batteries for our smoke alarms and locking up cleaning materials and medicines *now*. The quiz was a great reminder."

Although the lists of scary stats, safety steps, and action items in this chapter may seem a little overwhelming, the goal is simply to focus your efforts on key areas. Safety precautions aren't exactly exciting, but they are effective.

The Basics

After your youngest child is past the toddler stage, you probably won't need to keep the baby gates up and you can remove the padding from the corners of the coffee table. But there are many other precautions throughout the home to remember:

- **On every floor:** Install smoke and carbon monoxide detectors and check them once a month. When you reset the clocks in the fall and spring, change detector batteries, too—it's an easy way to remember. Also, keep a fire extinguisher in the kitchen and by any stairs. Plan fire escape routes with your children and practice "stop, drop, and roll" in case clothing catches on fire. Keep electrical cords out of children's reach.
- **By the window:** Tie up cords from window blinds, especially if the blinds aren't the new child-safe variety. Install window guards to prevent falls (but be sure they can be removed easily in case of fire). Never place climbable furniture under or near a window.
- **On sliding glass doors:** Place decals at your child's eye level so they can see they're not open and don't crash into or through them.
- **On the floor:** Secure all rugs and carpets to avoid slips and trips. Use nonskid backing under throw rugs. If you have

children under age 3, vacuum often; anytime you see coins, paper clips, or buttons on the floor, pick them up instantly. Remember, any small object can become a choking hazard.

- **In the bedroom:** Bunk beds are fun, but they're not safe for kids under 5. Regularly check bunk beds to make sure they are secure and stable: A wobbly structure could collapse on a child. And *never* allow jumping on a bunk bed.

- **In the bathroom:** Stick nonskid strips in the tub. Warn children about the dangers of electrocution, and keep electrical appliances like hair dryers unplugged and out of reach.

- **On the hot water heater:** To avoid scalding burns, set the temperature at a safe level—between 120°F and 125°F, or 49°C to 52°C.

- **In the kitchen:** Turn pot handles away from front edges to avoid burns. Always supervise older children when they are working in the kitchen, especially while they're using knives or the stove.

- **In a locked cabinet:** If you *must* have a gun in the home, store it unloaded and locked out of reach. Store ammunition in a different location.

- **By the phone:** Keep a list of emergency numbers next to the telephone. Include 911, poison control (1-800-222-1222), your pediatrician, and a close neighbor. It's also a good idea to list your own address and phone number, which kids or visitors could easily forget in a crisis.

Careful Training

On the road to adulthood, kids will face many risks; showing them ways to avoid injuries is like giving them an invisible suit of armor. As with the other healthy habits covered so far, use the 4 Is—identify, inform, instruct, and instill.

1. **Identify.** Evaluate your child's current safety habits and identify what needs to change.
2. **Inform.** Explain the most common risks and how to avoid them.
3. **Instruct.** Teach them NOT to overlook, underestimate, or ignore dangerous situations. Train them NOT to be careless.
4. **Instill.** This is extra important, because kids seem to take more risks when you're not around. Do your best to make sure your child's safety habits are virtually automatic.

What Increases the Likelihood of an Accident

- A major life change, such as a death in the family, a chronic illness, or a move
- A significant change in your child's usual routine
- Lack of familiarity with surroundings—being on vacation, visiting friends, staying with relatives
- Being rushed, stressed, or overtired
- Being distracted and unsupervised
- Being caught in crowded conditions

Evaluating Your Current Safety Habits

One of the best parts of being a kid is having time to speed around on bikes, toss the football, or play water games in the pool. Kids can work their bodies pretty hard, but they're not indestructible. The causes and consequences of injuries vary depending on your child's age and developmental level. Let's look back at the RealAge Healthy Kids Test to find out how your family's safety habits scored.

 In a personal vehicle, does your child sit in a car seat or booster seat with the seat belt fastened correctly?

Automobile accidents are the number one cause of death among children. Promise yourself that you will never allow kids to ride in your car without being properly restrained—not even for a few feet! Children quickly learn that this is a nonnegotiable precaution. Kids are at huge risk of severe injury or even death if they're not properly restrained with—depending on their age and size—a child safety seat, booster seat, or properly fitted lap/shoulder belt.

One big problem, however, is that many well-intentioned parents don't manage to install seats properly. Perhaps you've already discovered how tricky this can be, thanks to the wide range of car models, seat belt configurations, and safety seat designs. However, the resulting statistics are frightening: only 20 percent of families use car seats correctly, and fewer than 10 percent use booster seats correctly.

Wondering whether your child's car seat is properly installed and if you are using it correctly? Visit a car seat inspection station. Check with the National Highway Traffic Safety Administration website to find one near you. Or call 1-888-327-4236 or 1-866-SEATCHECK or go to www.seatcheck.org.

Choosing the Right Car Seat

During an accident or even an abrupt stop or sharp curve, safety restraints work by stopping your child's body as the car slows, reducing the forces on the body and preventing contact with hard surfaces inside the vehicle, other occupants, and with dangers outside the car, such as the road or other vehicles.

Children who are either under 12 months or who weigh under 20 pounds should always ride in a rear-facing car seat—so a 10-month-old who weighs 23 pounds should face the rear, as should a 13-month-old who weighs 18 pounds. Be sure that your car seat is suitable for your child's weight—many hold children up to 35 pounds. The backseat is the safest place for a child to sit.

Children over age 1 who weigh 20 to 40 pounds can ride in a forward-facing car seat. There are also combination forward-facing car-booster seats with harness straps for kids who weigh up to 65 pounds. These are significantly safer than a regular booster seat that uses the car's lap-shoulder belt. Once children are tall enough—about 4'9"—they can be properly protected by a regular seat belt. (Most kids reach this height between 8 and 12 years old.) Children no longer need a booster seat when they meet these three requirements:

1. **Placement.** The shoulder belt fits across the middle of their shoulder and chest, and doesn't cut into the neck or throat.
2. **Fit.** The lap belt fits snugly across their thighs, not across the stomach.
3. **Position.** They can sit comfortably against the seat back, knees bent and feet hanging down.

  Seat Belt Safety

Whether your child needs a booster seat or is tall enough to ride without one, be sure that he or she always uses the shoulder belt properly, not behind their back or under their arm.

Help older kids understand a little of the science behind seat belts. During an accident the safety belt spreads the crash forces over a broad area of the body, distributing them evenly to the body's larger, stronger areas, such as the chest, hips, and shoulders. A safety belt also allows a person to stop as the car is stopping, so the wearer can "ride down" the crash.

As always, kids tend to mimic the behavior of

A front-seat passenger is 30 percent more likely to be injured or killed in a car crash than passengers in a rear seat.

those around them—that means you. So set a good example by using seat belts correctly yourself.

If you establish car safety habits early, wearing seat belts will become a normal practice for life, used in every instance and in every vehicle. Which is just what you want.

Does your child sit in the backseat of the vehicle?

As I've mentioned, the backseat is the safest place for a child of any age to ride, whether the vehicle has airbags or not. The lives of thousands of children have been saved solely because they were sitting in the backseat, according to recent studies.

Sure, the front seat is alluring. Kids like to sit there because they can see better and they have easier access to you and the radio. But don't give in. Children (especially those under age 12) should always ride in the backseat. Statistics show that this can help avoid neck or spine injuries in the event of a sudden stop or crash.

 ### If your child drives, how confident are you about his/her skills behind the wheel?

It can be pretty darn scary when children start to drive. In fact, this is one of the milestones that parents fear most. With reason. The risk of crashes is higher among teenagers than any other age group.

So even if you are relatively confident of your child's driving skills, supervise car use carefully during the first few years of driving. It takes a while to master the rules of the road. Provide as much behind-the-wheel driving practice with you as possible. This will help instill a better understanding of and respect for the dynamics and power of a motor vehicle. It will also allow you to point out some of the mistakes other drivers commonly make and talk about anticipating what other drivers are about to do. New drivers often are so focused on their own driving that they fail to notice other drivers' actions.

Regular reminders about following safe-driving rules are a good idea, even if you start to feel like a nag. Seat belt use tends to decline quite a bit during teenage years, especially among boys, so emphasize that everyone in the car must wear a seat belt on every trip, even short trips.

Until new drivers are sufficiently skilled, limit the number of passengers your teen can have in the car. The risk of fatal injury for a 16- or 17-year-old driver has been shown to increase with the number of passengers. Even having just one other teenager in the front seat can make a teen driver more careless.

Other passengers aren't the only distractions for teens behind the wheel. Talking on a cell phone, fiddling with the CD player, fussing with their hair, eating—all can lead to accidents. Using a cell phone without a hands-free device also is illegal in many states. Remind teen drivers to remain

Are SUVs safer?

No. Despite their size and bulk, it appears that children in SUVs are no better protected than those in ordinary cars. However, silver cars may be safer, regardless of the style. One study found that silver cars are as much as 50 percent less likely to be involved in serious accidents than cars of other colors. Researchers speculate that their lighter, more reflective shade may make silver cars more visible on the road.

Lay Down the Rules and Reduce Accidents

Teens whose parents have clear rules about who and how many people are allowed to ride with them are less likely to be distracted by friends, get a ticket, drive too fast, or drive aggressively. Ask them every time:

- **Who's** going with you?
- **What** can't you forget to do (buckle up)?
- **Where** are you going?
- **When** will you be home?

If the answers don't fit your rules, don't hand over the keys until they do.

focused on the road at all times so they can react quickly and drive defensively. Talk with all your children—even nondrivers—about how multiple passengers and other distractions can lead to accidents.

  Parked Car Dangers

Even on a relatively cool day, if the sun is shining, the temperature inside a parked car can spike to life-threatening levels in fifteen to thirty minutes. Never leave children (or animals) alone in a parked car, especially on a sunny day. And heat isn't the only danger: Children as old as 14 have been known to climb into the driver's seat, pop the trunk, hop out of the car, and climb into the trunk. Some are curious, while others are simply looking for a clever place to hide during a game of tag or hide-and-seek. This can be fatal. Children die in car trunks from heat or suffocation. Take these simple steps to prevent this tragedy:

1. **Lock up.** Keep your car locked with the trunk closed, even when it's parked at home.
2. **Hide 'em.** Keep car keys where children cannot get to them.
3. **Keep watch.** Don't send kids out to play and assume they'll be fine; check on them regularly.
4. **Stay together.** Take kids into stores with you, even for a quick errand.
5. **Attach a latch.** If your car does not have an interior trunk-release mechanism, contact your dealer to get one retrofitted.

Also beware of other items that kids can climb into and get trapped. Those old refrigerators, freezers, and extra-large cool-ers that may be kicking around the garage, basement, or yard can be extremely dangerous. A child who climbs into one and gets trapped can suffocate in fewer than ten minutes.

  Does your child wear appropriate protective gear (helmet, elbow and knee pads, mouth guards, etc.) when participating in activities or sports?

Getting kids to wear protective gear gets harder as kids get older. Many parents say they have a tough time maintaining this habit once their kids hit adolescence because they think it's uncool, uncomfortable, unnecessary, or all three. In fact, recent studies show that most teens don't wear bike helmets, even if required by law, and very few wear helmets when skateboarding, snowboarding, or skiing. In addition, kids wear protective gear far less than many parents think they do—once they're out of sight of adults, off go the helmets and pads.

Reasons for NOT Wearing Protective Equipment	How to Respond
"It isn't cool."	Join forces with other parents to make the habit more widely practiced; add favorite stickers or painted images to the gear.
"It's uncomfortable, annoying, or hot."	Get equipment that fits properly; it won't help much or at all if it doesn't.
"I'm only practicing/fooling around."	Let kids know that these are the times when most accidents happen.
"I'm staying close to home."	
"*You* don't wear one."	Always wear protective gear yourself.
"I don't need it."	Show kids shots of pros who wear the gear.

Given this research, ask your children how often they wear their protective gear. If they answer "sometimes" or "never," find out why they don't wear it all the time. Identifying the reason(s) can help you figure out how to change this habit.

Kids often say, "I don't need a helmet. I've been skateboarding since I was 4." This false sense of security is something you need to watch out for. Make sure your kids understand that experience is no protection since injuries happen at all skill levels. Many kids think that once they've mastered a sport or activity, they're invincible.

Also, there are dangers that kids have absolutely no control over: the distracted motorist who doesn't see them on their bikes, the baseball that's hit straight at a kid's head, or the newbie skater who crashes and takes down five other skaters in the process. No amount of experience can prevent the unpredictable actions of others.

Strap on That Helmet

If you've decided to pick your battles and focus on getting your child to wear just one piece of equipment, make it a helmet. Hands down, the head is the most important body part to protect. While most cuts, bruises, and broken bones will heal, head injuries are often permanent and disabling. They can lead to a loss of certain neurological functions and, in serious cases, victims can lapse into a coma and die. Scary stuff.

You definitely want a helmet to absorb any blows to your child's

Who Wears Helmets?

- More girls than boys
- Half of kids 5 to 9
- About a third of kids 10 to 14.

Helmets can prevent over 80 percent of head and brain injuries, so be sure your child is putting one on.

head—that means one lined with thick plastic foam (firm polystyrene) to cushion the skull. A good helmet can reduce the risk of head and brain injury by as much as 88 percent.

When to Wear One

Because more childhood injuries are associated with bicycles than anything else except car accidents, wearing a helmet while cycling should be nonnegotiable. Sixty percent of serious bike-related injuries are head injuries. Helmets are also a must for skateboarding, skiing, ice skating, in-line skating, etc. A crash or fall can change a child's life forever if his head hits the street, sidewalk, curb, lamppost, car, tree, etc. A fall of only two feet can cause a skull fracture or brain injury.

> Head injuries are the leading cause of bike-related deaths.

Save Your Kids from iPoditis

Using earbud headphones may let your kids listen to tunes at a higher volume without your yelling, "Turn it down!" They also fit nicely under a helmet. But whether the sounds are hip-hop or Barney, overexposure can harm sensitive hearing mechanisms in their ears.

To keep kids' hearing sharp for years to come, noise researchers recommend limiting kids' earbud use to no more than an hour a day and keeping the volume no higher than 90 decibels (about the sound of a vacuum cleaner or lawn mower).

You can download free software at apple.com that locks in a volume limit on your child's iPod.

Finding the Perfect Fit

Helmets lose almost all of their power to protect if they don't fit properly, so take some time choosing one. Besides, kids won't wear them if they slip, pinch, fall over their eyes, or are so

**You Know You've Chosen
the Right Helmet If . . .**

- **It's snug.** There's no slipping from side to side or front to back.
- **It's level.** It sits square on top of the head, covering the top of the forehead with its front edge two finger-widths above the eyebrows. It shouldn't tilt in any direction.
- **It's stable.** The chin strap is double insurance that the helmet won't slip or come off in a fall. The strap should be snug when your child opens his mouth. (One finger should fit between the chin and chin strap when the mouth is closed.)
- **It's certified.** The helmet should be labeled on the inside as approved by the U.S. Consumer Product Safety Commission (CPSC).

tight that they produce an instant headache. Once you've found a good fit for your child, insist that it's worn correctly. Children tend to wear helmets tilted or with the straps dangling, which renders the head gear useless.

Encouraging Helmet Use

Kids are more likely to wear a helmet if they like the way it looks, so let them help pick it out. Head to the bike store for printed covers in a wide range of patterns that slip over the outside of helmets. Some even look like shark's fins or have dinosaur scales. There are also multipurpose helmets that can be worn for bicycling, skating, or skiing.

Of course, your child is much more likely to wear a helmet if you do. The stats prove it. One study found that 67 percent of children wore helmets when adult riders with them did. But only 50 percent of kids wore them when their adult companions didn't. Unfortunately, parents don't wear helmets more than 60 percent of the time. (If they knew that wearing a helmet every time they cycled could make their RealAge as much as one year younger, perhaps more parents would!)

The Extreme Risk of Extreme Sports

Many kids are attracted to the adrenaline rush of "extreme" sports—aggressive, trick-filled skateboarding, skating, and snowboarding. You may have noticed skateboard parks popping up in your own community, often with dramatic ramps and half-pipes. It's a big competitive sport.

Unfortunately, injuries from roller sports—skateboarding, in-line and roller skating, and scooters—have increased along with their popularity. Each year, more than 297,000 children ages 5 to 14 end up needing medical treatment as a result of roller-sport injuries. Here's the breakdown:

- The most serious injury is head trauma, so a helmet is an absolute must.
- The wrist and forearm are the most common fracture sites, so when you buy skates, buy wrist guards.
- Add elbow and knee pads to help kids avoid fractures and dislocations—they cut wrist and elbow injuries by about 85 percent and knee injuries by 32 percent.

How to Fall Gracefully

It may seem counterintuitive to teach your child how to fall when the point of most sports is to remain upright. But falls happen all the time, especially when learning a new sport, so help your child practice falling techniques—they may reduce the chances of serious injury. The basics:

- Crouch down if you feel yourself losing your balance, so you won't have as far to fall.
- Don't try to break the fall with your hands—you may break both wrists. Instead, try to land on the fleshy parts of the body and roll.
- Relax your body rather than stiffening up.

If your child does tricks or plays roller hockey, make sure he or she wears heavy-duty gear.

School Sports and Activities

As mentioned in Chapter 3, school sports help kids build valuable skills—self-discipline, sportsmanship, leadership, socialization, and more. Unfortunately, school sports are the second most frequent cause of injury for both boys and girls, especially adolescents. Whether it's a feeling of invincibility or impulsivity, most student athletes opt out of wearing even simple knee pads and shin guards, leaving them vulnerable to painful and disabling injuries.

Have you ever been kicked in the shins with a cleat? Ouch!

But the last thing most teenagers want is to look different from their peers, and wearing pads and a helmet when no one else is does exactly that. So work with other parents and coaches to make protective gear mandatory. It will help keep everyone free from injuries on the field or court. That's a win.

 ### Water, Water, Everywhere

Most kids find water irresistible. Whether it's crashing waves or a kiddie pool, splashing around can provide hours of amusement. However, because even shallow water can be dangerous, reducing the risk of water accidents is very important. A child can drown in less than an inch of water.

Is your child monitored while taking a bath?

Your child may view bath time as the highlight of the day or as cruel and unusual punishment. Either way, keep safety in mind since the risk potential is real. There are way too many drownings and scaldings among young children. Always keep a close eye on kids under age 6 while they bathe. This means staying within arm's reach. Make sure babysitters follow this rule, too. (More safety pointers for sitters are at the end of this chapter.) Simply checking in on them every now and then won't suffice; children can drown quietly in just a few minutes.

Also, don't mistake a baby bath seat as a safety device. Babies can climb out of them and drown.

Scalding water can cause serious burns that require painful treatment and may result in scarring, physical and emotional disability, and years of skin graft surgeries. Luckily, nearly 75 percent of these injuries are preventable. Keep young children away from the faucet and regularly remind them not to touch faucet handles. Also, buy soft, insulated covers for the bathtub faucets. They're good safeguards against accidental burns or bumps. As kids get older, teach them to always run the cold water first and then add hot water, and to always turn off the hot water before the cold. Show older children and babysitters how to test the bath water temperature by putting their elbow in first. If the water feels hot on their elbow, it could burn them.

As mentioned earlier, keeping the hot water heater set between 120°F and 125°F (49°C to 52°C) can help avoid serious burns.

Water hazards are everywhere around the home, not just in the bathroom. Babies under age 1 can and do fall headfirst into toilets and buckets and drown. Empty and overturn water containers when you have finished using them; keep doors to bathrooms and laundry rooms closed and toilet seats down.

Does your child know how to swim?

When the sun comes out and the weather heats up, many families head to the pool or the beach. You want your child to love swimming and splashing, but you also want to make sure that water fun is safe.

> For children ages 1 to 4, most drownings happen in swimming pools.

Ages 0–5—never leave 'em alone. Although swimming programs are available for babies and young children, these classes focus on building confidence and encouraging children to enjoy the water, not teaching them how to swim. Four-year-olds usually have the mind/body skills needed for formal swimming instruction and water safety training. Still, even if your youngster can swim, don't rely on beginner skills. Tragedy can happen quickly. Getting engrossed in a good book, a good conversation, or just making a quick run to the bathroom is enough time for a child to slip under quietly. Most children who drown in a home swimming pool were out of sight of an adult for fewer than five minutes. Also, inflatable inner tubes, floaties, and water wings are toys, not safety devices. Watch kids constantly.

For every child who drowns, three others require emergency care. Of these, more than 40 percent are hospitalized. Water immersion injuries can cause brain damage and long-term disabilities, ranging from memory problems to a vegetative state.

Into the Wild Blue Water

If water play involves lakes, rivers, and oceans, make sure your child stays within the designated swimming area or, if a beach has lifeguards, in sight of the lifeguard tower.

An unpredictable danger with ocean swimming is rip currents, which typically occur when changes in the ocean floor force waves back out to sea with unusual force. Rip currents can drag people out with them, and it's easy to panic when swimmers realize they're not strong enough to fight the current.

Teach kids what to do in a rip

Water Safety Rules Every Kid Needs to Know

- Never run near a swimming pool.
- Never push or jump on others around water.
- Never swim alone.
- Jump into water feet first rather than head-first if water is shallow (5 to 6 feet or less).
- If you believe you even *might* be in trouble, immediately call or wave for help.
- Follow pool rules and lifeguard directions.

current: Swim parallel to the beach, and don't even try to swim straight back to the shore until you see people swimming normally farther down the beach. If you grow tired, wave to signal that you are having trouble. When you do get back to shore, alert the lifeguard and other swimmers of the rip current.

If boating is on your family's agenda, provide life jackets approved by the U.S. Coast Guard for all children. Also use these life jackets if your child participates in water sports like rafting or tubing.

Sun Safety

All pediatricians have treated really bad sunburns, sometimes on babies who can't even walk yet, let alone apply sunblock. And not just in summertime, in the winter and even on cloudy days. Overexposure to UV rays from the sun during childhood and adolescence doesn't just cause painful sunburns, blistering, and peeling; it greatly increases the risk of skin cancer as an adult—particularly melanoma, the deadliest form of skin cancer. Multiple studies have linked blistering sunburns in childhood to melanoma later in life.

About 50 to 80 Percent of a Lifetime of Sun Damage Happens During Childhood

Long, sunny days sound like the stuff a kid's dreams are made of. But in a given year, kids get three times more sun exposure than adults, leaving them vulnerable to developing skin cancer later on.

Sunscreen with an SPF of *at least* 30 is a must and should be worn all the time outdoors, on the beach and off. Ditto for hats and sunglasses—young scalps and eyes are at risk, too.

Follow these steps to protect delicate young skin:

- Put a hat on your child and cover up as much skin as possible. Lightweight clothing doesn't provide much sun protection, so your child may still need sunscreen underneath.

- Apply PABA-free sunscreen with an SPF of at least 30 to children and babies. Reapply every few hours and always after swimming.
- Have kids wear sunglasses with UV protection starting at a young age.
- Limit direct exposure to the sun between the hours of 10 a.m. and 3 p.m., when the UV rays are the most intense.

Keep children out of direct sun whenever possible, especially babies under 6 months. Seek out shady locations where kids can play out of the heat and sun.

RealAge Projection: **Children who get into the habit of limiting sun exposure now are likely to stick with this healthy habit as adults. If they do, their RealAge could be 29 when they are actually 32.**

Choking

For young kids, especially babies under 12 months, choking is one of the most common causes of accidental death.

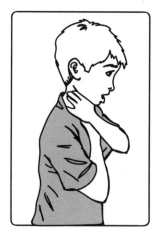

Have you taught your child the universal choking sign?
A number of things make small children more vulnerable to choking than adults: small upper airways, inexperience with chewing, and their tendency to put anything and everything in their mouths. Because every child is at risk of choking from food and other

objects, every child should be taught the universal choking signal pictured on page 222.

Teach kids to place both hands across the front of their throat, crossed at the wrists. This gesture should be taken as a serious sign that your child cannot breathe.

Check with local hospitals and American Red Cross chapters for classes that teach choking rescue techniques and other critical life-saving skills.

 ### Choking and Children Under 1

Babies naturally put things in their mouths, which is cute if they are chewing on a large stuffed toy or their own fingers. But it's dangerous if they swallow or inhale something small such as marbles, peanuts, or small toys belonging to older siblings. For toys, a good rule of thumb is to avoid items that fit through a cardboard toilet-paper tube.

Take the following preventive steps:

- **Think small.** Be vigilant about keeping small objects out of your baby's reach. This includes small chunks of food.
- **Sit for meals.** When your baby begins to eat solid foods, be sure she sits upright while eating.

Beware of Balloons

Many parents are surprised to learn that balloons are a leading cause of childhood death. The danger lies in a swallowed balloon taking the shape of the child's windpipe or airway rather than moving down it as a solid object would. Children through age 8 are at risk, so keep a close eye on those party balloons. Put uninflated or popped balloons far out of children's reach. You may want to avoid latex rubber balloons altogether and use mylar balloons instead—they don't deflate or pop as easily as latex balloons, so they are less of a hazard.

Common Foods That Can Cause Choking

- Nuts
- Spoonfuls of peanut butter
- Hot dogs
- Chunks of meat and poultry
- Chunks of cheese
- White bread
- Raw vegetables (carrots, celery, lettuce)
- Whole grapes
- Hard candy
- Popcorn
- Snack chips

- **Consider age.** Choose toys that are age-appropriate. If your baby is given toys for older ages, store them safely out of reach until she's the right age.
- **Don't toy around.** Tell older children, siblings, or visitors to keep small toys away from the baby.

Choking and Children Ages 1 to 4

Always supervise small children who are eating finger foods, being sure they stay sitting upright. Don't hurry eating. Put only a small amount of food on the tray at a time. Also, make sure the pieces of food are small—ideally no more than one-half inch in any direction. If you're not sure, err on the small side. Cut meat across the grain into small pieces so it's easier to chew.

Besides small toys and marbles, keep items suchs as pen caps, small batteries, and coins away from young children. Do a sofa-cushion dig periodically to check for choking hazards that have fallen through the cracks. Get down on the floor from time to time and look around at a baby's eye level for any hazards you might not see at adult height.

> #### Finger Food Fun
>
> Here are some safe finger foods.
>
> - Cooked carrots, cut lengthwise—not in circles
> - Wheat toast with crusts removed
> - Scrambled eggs
> - O-shaped cereals
> - Peas, cooked until soft (no pods)
> - Avocados
> - Cooked pasta
> - Bananas and pear pieces, ripe and soft

Poison Proofing Your Home

While on the topic of kids putting things in their mouths, let's talk common household items that are poisonous to children—keeping in mind that if something's accessible, kids will taste it. This list includes dishwashing detergent, plants, liquor, holiday ornaments, cat litter and excrement, all kinds of household cleansers, vitamins, medications—both prescription and OTC—and more.

It's really important to keep toxic substances out of kids' reach. Store them in high cabinets, not under the sink; use cupboard locks and lockable cases; and purchase containers with child-resistant tops. But know that by 18 months (sometimes earlier) a child can open many containers, and by age 3, some children may be able to pop off those child-resistant tops—even if you can't.

Check every room for potential poisons. Don't overlook the living room and bedrooms. Also, remember that some substances that aren't toxic for adults are for children. For example, alcohol can poison

Common but Dangerous

Some of these items may not seem risky at first, but all can be hazardous to a child:

- Over-the-counter medicines such as cold and flu treatments
- Creams and ointments
- Vitamins
- Gardening products
- Perfumes
- Alcohol
- Car products
- Cigarette butts

children and lead to seizures, coma, and even death. Remove not only wine and liquor but also products that contain alcohol, such as mouthwashes, aftershaves, and colognes—and check handbags and briefcases too, especially if you carry toiletries and medicines with you.

Studies show that most poisonings occur when a substance is left on a bench or counter after use. So think ahead. If you are scrubbing the sink and the doorbell rings, take the cleanser with you. If you've half-finished a beer and don't want the rest, don't leave the bottle on a table. Never turn your back on a child who's near a dangerous-to-them product.

Poisoning from Vitamins

Many parents don't realize that one of the most common causes of childhood poisoning in the home is something you and your children may ingest every day: vitamins. Formulas that contain iron are responsible for 30 percent of children's deaths from poisoning. So be sure to keep all vitamins out of children's reach and never refer to them as "candy." Young children might think it's okay to eat a handful of brightly colored vitamins—and this could have fatal consequences.

How to Tell If Your Child Has Been Poisoned

It can be tricky to tell when children have swallowed a poisonous substance, especially if they're too young to talk. Pay close attention if you suspect this has happened. Signs that children may have ingested a poison include the following:

- They can't follow you with their eyes, or their eyes go around in circles.
- They are sleepy before it's nap time or bedtime.
- They suddenly throw up.
- They have burns around the lips and mouth.
- They have stains around the lips and mouth.
- Their breath suddenly smells foul.

Also, look for telltale evidence, like an open container within reach or a spilled bottle of pills.

If You Think Your Child Has Been Poisoned

Keep calm. If you know what your child swallowed, look on the container for first-aid instructions.

Post this number by your phone: 1-800-222-1222. An operator will connect you to the nearest poison control center. Or call 911 or your doctor. Provide your child's age, height, and weight. If you know, explain how your child was exposed to the poison: Was it swallowed? Splashed in the eyes? Inhaled? If you know what the poisonous substance was, take the container to the phone with you and provide the label information.

Follow the instructions from the poison center or your doctor carefully.

By the way, one classic bit of advice about poisonings has changed: Don't bother keeping a bottle of syrup of ipecac on hand. This induces vomiting, and in many cases vomiting can cause more harm than good. For instance, it can cause complications with corrosive chemicals that burn on the way down and again on the way up.

 Keep an Eye on Older Kids

Although poisoning is less likely among older kids, those pretty pills on the medicine cabinet shelves can tempt teens. Abuse of prescription medications among teens is rising at an alarming rate, and many teens think that if a family member takes something, it must be safe. Recreational use can be the gateway to addiction, overdose, or worse. To reduce the risk of prescription pilfering, talk openly with your kids about the dangers of drugs—and dispose of medications you no longer need.

> Prescription drug abuse ranks second in illicit drug use among children in the United States, after marijuana.

RealAge Projection: Getting into the habit of taking too many medications or taking them improperly is dangerous for all children. If they continue misusing prescription or OTC medications as adults, it could age them almost 5 years. That means at 35, they'll look and feel like they're 40.

Keeping Medications Safe

- Close medicine containers immediately after using them, then put them in a safe place, out of the reach of children of all ages.
- Keep medicines in their original containers.
- Keep drugs out of sight of children.
- Don't leave medicines on a countertop or bedside table.
- If a medication has expired, throw it away.

Powerful prescription pain relievers, stimulants, sedatives, and tranquilizers are finding their way out of family medicine cabinets and into schools and "pharming" parties where children share, swap, and swallow prescription drugs. Although open and honest dialogue about the dangers of drugs greatly reduces your child's risk of abuse and addiction, peer pressure can be persuasive. Limit the temptation in your own home by securing all medications in a place that's safe from your children and their friends.

Also, be aware that many popular and potent drugs, such as Vicodin, OxyContin, and Valium, are easily obtained online. Often referred to as "pill mills," unregulated, unscrupulous overseas websites will sell pills to anyone with a credit card. So monitor your child's online activity (and your credit card, too).

Expecting the Unexpected

So you've taken all the steps to make your children as safe as possible, eliminating potential hazards within the home and protecting as much as possible against those that can happen away from it. But face it, accidents still happen. The key to handling them is being well prepared. The next few questions from the test focus on how ready your family is for an emergency.

Is there a first-aid kit in your home?

Even the safest households have their share of bumps, scrapes, and stings. When your child comes running to you with an injury, you should have a first-aid kit within easy reach—not just a box of bandages and some all-purpose ointment stuck in the corner of the medicine cabinet.

Your first-aid kit should be clean, handy (not buried in the garage or basement), and well stocked. If your knowledge of first aid is a little sketchy, sign up for a class in your community. Basic first-aid training can be very beneficial in small or big emergency situations—and in today's world, these can happen anywhere. Many classes also teach cardiopulmonary resuscitation (CPR), which is a particularly valuable skill to know when you have children.

Because emergencies can also easily happen in the car, and because we spend so much time driving with kids, it's smart to keep one kit in your home, one in every car, and to take one with you on vacations, as kids are more likely to have accidents in unfamiliar surroundings. That way you're able to handle an emergency at a moment's notice. Whenever you use your kit, replace what you used as soon as possible so it's ready for the next time.

Involve your children in preparing a family emergency plan. Once your kids are old enough, work with them to collect the resources needed to meet basic needs during an emergency—hurricanes, floods, wildfires, tornadoes, blizzards, or manmade calamities. As a rule, when kids feel prepared, they cope better.

Clear the Air

Nowadays, air within homes and other buildings can contain more dangerous pollutants than the air outdoors. Given that

What Should Be in Your First-Aid Kit

- 4" × 4" gauze pads
- 8" × 10" gauze pads
- One package of 2" gauze roll bandages
- Box of assorted adhesive bandages
- Tylenol for pain relief
- Benadryl or other antihistamine for allergic reactions
- Adhesive tape
- Latex gloves
- Sealed moistened towelettes
- Antibiotic ointment
- Disposable instant ice bags
- Scissors
- Tweezers
- Thermometer in a protective case
- Activated charcoal for poisoning—call Poison Control Center BEFORE using
- At least one blanket
- Plastic bag
- Emergency first-aid handbook

Additional supplies to have on hand for emergencies*

- Three-day supply of clean water—allow 1 gallon per person per day
- Three-day supply of nonperishable food such as canned meats, canned fruits and vegetables, energy bars, juice, and baby food
- Manual can opener
- Battery-operated radio and extra batteries
- Flashlights and extra batteries
- Fire extinguisher
- Matches in a waterproof container
- Toothbrushes, toothpaste, soap, other toiletries

*For an exhaustive list, please visit www.redcross.org.

most people spend approximately 90 percent of their time indoors, this is unnerving. Fortunately, indoor air pollution is one risk that you can do a lot about. For starters, be sure your home is:

- Tested for lead
- Tested for radon
- Equipped with smoke detectors
- Equipped with carbon monoxide detectors

RealAge Projection: **Being exposed to environmental toxins is dangerous for children's health, both short- and long-term. If you fail to protect them now and they don't take precautions later, they could age themselves by as many as 3 years.**

Get the Lead Out

Lead poisoning is one of the most serious environmental health threats children face at home, and it can do harm before anyone knows it because the symptoms aren't immediately obvious. Exposure to lead can cause permanent learning and behavioral problems, damage hearing, and harm the nervous system, including the brain. A blood test is the only way to detect it. Most local health clinics offer this test free. Your pediatrician should do routine lead screening and testing at regular check-ups.

Although the use of lead-based paints in homes was banned decades ago, the danger is still present in some older buildings. If your dwelling was built before 1978—and especially before 1950—have it checked for lead-based paint. Your local or state health department can tell you how to have your home, soil, or water tested. There is usually little or no cost associated with these tests, and inexpensive lead testing kits are available at most hardware stores.

If you discover lead paint in your home, don't attempt to remove it yourself. Removal requires professional training in handling hazardous materials to control and contain lead dust.

Radon

Radon is a radioactive gas that is invisible, odorless, tasteless—and causes cancer. It is a natural by-product of uranium in soil, rock, and water, and it can get into the air you and your kids breathe. Unlike lead, it doesn't matter how old your home is; both old and new homes can contain radon. There are inexpensive devices available for measuring radon at the hardware store; check with your local health department for more information on testing and removal.

Carbon Monoxide

Another deadly gas that can be released in your home is carbon monoxide (CO). You can't see or smell it, which makes it even more dangerous. Carbon monoxide poisons more than 2,110 children age 5 and younger each year. While everyone is at risk,

The *Other* Kind of Smoke Danger

Here's an air pollutant you won't need to test for: tobacco smoke. If there's a smoker in the home, your kids are breathing this toxin. Whether it comes from a cigarette, pipe, or cigar, tobacco smoke contains at least forty compounds that are known to cause cancer.

Besides cancer, children who are exposed to tobacco smoke have an increased risk of pneumonia, bronchitis, asthma, coughing, wheezing, excess phlegm, and ear infections. Newborns also have an increased risk of SIDS.

For the sake of your children's health (as well as your own), please don't smoke. And don't let guests smoke either.

Potential Sources of CO Poisoning

Besides installing a carbon monoxide detector, check these potential sources of CO poisoning and have them professionally serviced regularly:

Furnaces

- Check filters and filtering systems for blockages and dirt.
- Have a professional check for high concentrations of CO in the flue gases or cracks in the combustion chamber.
- Look at the ignition system. If the flame is mostly yellow in a natural gas-fired furnace, this may be a sign that fuel is not burning completely and releasing excess CO.

Venting systems to the outside: flues, chimneys, and gas clothes dryer vents

- Check chimneys for nests that may block gas from escaping.
- Check flues and chimneys for cracks, corrosion, holes, and debris.
- Check outside dryer vents for lint buildup.

Appliances that use flammable fuels such as oil, wood, kerosene, or natural gas

- These can include clothes dryers, kitchen ranges, ovens, and water heaters.
- Check pilot lights since malfunctions can release CO inside the home. Monitor gas stoves and ovens closely.

Space heaters

- Check to make sure these are vented properly.

Barbecue grills and generators

- Do not use these indoors.
- Do not use these in an attached garage, even with the door open.
- Do not use these outside in front of an open window.

infants and children are the most vulnerable. The initial symptoms of CO poisoning—headache, nausea, dizziness, chest pain—mimic other illnesses, so it's difficult to diagnose. Sleeping children can become ill or die without ever waking up to complain of symptoms. Protect your family by installing inexpensive CO sensors on every level and in every bedroom of your home and testing them regularly.

Create a plan of action for your kids to follow if the alarm does go off. Stress the importance of leaving the house immediately, and agree on a meeting place outdoors where you can breathe fresh air. Do not call for help until you've left the building.

Smoke

Few things are scarier than a burning house. That's why smoke alarms are essential. Install at least one on each floor of your home. Check them monthly and replace the batteries twice a year. A simple way to remember to do this is to change the batteries when you change the clocks each spring and fall.

It's important to work out a fire escape plan with your children. Show them two ways out of the house in case one is blocked by fire. Teach them to feel a door for heat before opening it to be sure the exit is safe. Let your children know that no matter how frightening a fire might be, it's never okay to hide. Also, firefighters in all their gear may look spooky, so take a field trip to the local fire station to help kids get familiar with these local heroes, and pick up some tips about fire safety, too.

Where to Place Smoke Alarms

- On a ceiling or on a wall 6 to 12 inches below the ceiling
- Away from registers or air vents
- Away from areas with either a lot of or very little airflow (such as constantly opened doors or high peaks)

Set up a family meeting place, such as a neighbor's front yard, in case of fire. Rehearse the plan occasionally so that in the heat of an emergency your children will remember what to do.

Studies show that children may sleep through a smoke alarm. Test the alarm one night when the family's asleep to find out if this is a problem. In an emergency, you'll know who you need to wake up.

Safety Rules for Babysitters

Sitters may not be aware of these basic precautions. Give them a copy or post these on the refrigerator:

1. Never leave young children alone in the house or outside by themselves, even just for a minute. If children are under age 4, stay in the same room with them at all times.

2. Never let a young child near water (bathtub, swimming pool, even the toilet) without your supervision. It takes only a few inches of water and a few unsupervised moments for an infant or toddler to drown.

3. Never give any medication to a child without a parent's permission.

4. Never give children under age 4 nuts, popcorn, raw carrots, hard candy, or other small, hard foods that can be choked on. Always cut up hot dogs and grapes into small pieces before giving to young kids.

5. Never let a child play with plastic bags (they could suffocate) or with latex balloons and small toys that could be put into the mouth and choked on.

6. Never let children play on the stairs, near open windows or hot stoves, and around electrical outlets.

Avoid Overconfidence in Kids

Safety may not be the most exciting topic, but teaching kids to be safety-minded deserves the same attention as other health habits. Plenty of kids think, "Oh, that'll never happen to me," but, sadly, drowning, burns, scalding, head injuries, poisonings, electrocution, shootings, broken bones, and suffocation happen to kids every day.

Children who've never really been hurt and feel invincible are often the most vulnerable to accidents. Confidence is good, but overconfidence needs to be tempered. Be very direct about which situations pose risks and then pinpoint how to avoid these dangers.

Giving your children a realistic understanding of the risks outlined in this chapter can greatly reduce common accidents—the kind that study after study shows are avoidable.

Remember, if something is foreseeable, it is also preventable. With your guidance and gentle reminders about rules and limits, your kids will be safer as they grow and thrive.

What Your Babysitter Needs to Know About Your Child

Your Child

☐ Your child's routine:

☐ Mealtime _____

☐ Bath time _____

☐ Nap/bedtime _____

☐ Any special health information about your child (allergies and medication needs, for example)

_____

_____

☐ Fears and phobias

_____

_____

☐ Favorite and forbidden foods

_____

_____

Rules

☐ Your general house rules (i.e., no eating in the living room, homework before TV, only one hour of computer time, etc.)

_____

_____

_____

_____

☐ Child safety rules

_____

_____

☐ Rules for the babysitter such as no nonemergency phone calls, no visitors, limits on TV/computer time, whether or not they can leave the home

_____

_____

_____

Contact Information

☐ How to reach you in case of emergency and where you'll be (will you have a cell phone?)

_____

_____

☐ Emergency phone numbers such as poison control (1-800-222-1222) and 911

_____

_____

☐ Phone numbers for relatives, friends, and neighbors in case you can't be reached

☐ Name _____ Phone number _____

☐ Name _____ Phone number _____

☐ Child's doctors' names and contact information

☐ Name _____ Phone number _____

☐ Name _____ Phone number _____

☐ Insurance provider and policy #

_____

_____

_____

☐ Preferred hospital in case of emergency

_____

_____

_____

Where Things Are

☐ Location of smoke detectors, fire extinguishers, and exits from home in case of fire

_____

_____

_____

☐ Location of security system/alarms and how to work them

_____

_____

_____

☐ Location of door keys in case a child gets locked inside a room

_____

_____

_____

☐ Location of first-aid kit

_____

_____

_____

Chapter 8

CHECK UP
Staying on Top of Your Child's Health
(and preventing the illnesses that threaten kids most)

Even if you don't have a daughter, pretend for a moment that you do. Imagine her as a preteen. Sulking. Stubborn. Ignoring you. She doesn't want to go outside. Walk the dog. Go to dance practice. Take PE class. All she wants to do is sit and read, with headphones on, blocking out the world. When you actually make eye contact and suggest doing something active, you receive a glare. What do you do?

You don't want to pick a fight. And reading is hardly a bad thing. So you decide to do nothing.

Fast-forward twenty years. Imagine your child as a 32-year-old working mother. She still loves to read. But she's also self-conscious. She doesn't play Frisbee with her kids on the beach. She stays in the cabin when her family goes out snowboarding. And she most definitely doesn't dance or give toasts at weddings. Inside, she's sad about this, but feels she's not athletically inclined, and definitely not good with large groups.

Worse, she has just been diagnosed with type 2 diabetes. It's not curable, and it puts her at greater risk of heart disease, glaucoma, and kidney problems. In fact, her RealAge is 40– eight years older than her calendar age. You're surprised about the diabetes. She's not particularly heavy; just somewhat soft around the edges, as you might expect a 32-year-old mom to be. The thing is, getting diabetes as an adult has more to do with being sedentary and eating poorly than being overweight. And the two always seem to go hand in hand.

Let's focus a little more on type 2 diabetes. It's incurable, but it's also one of the most preventable of serious diseases. Yet the number of kids (and adults) who have it is soaring, but many parents don't know the difference between type 1 (not preventable) and type 2 (largely preventable). Take a look at the following chart that compares Jimmy and Timmy:

Jimmy—Has Type 1 Diabetes	Timmy—at Risk for Type 2 Diabetes
Age: **9**	Age: **9**
Height: **53 inches**	Height: **53 inches**
Weight: **65 pounds**	Weight: **85 pounds**
Type 1 characteristics • Also known as insulin-dependent or juvenile-onset diabetes, type 1 occurs when the pancreas produces too little insulin, the hormone that allows blood sugar (glucose) to be used as fuel. • Without enough insulin, glucose builds up dangerously in the bloodstream. • No cure	Type 2 characteristics • Also known as adult-onset or noninsulin-dependent diabetes, type 2 is preceded by insulin resistance, a condition where the body does not respond correctly to insulin. • Factors such as obesity, low physical activity, and a diet high in sugar and fat can make the body resist insulin's effects. • No cure

Jimmy—Has Type 1 Diabetes	Timmy—at Risk for Type 2 Diabetes
Why Jimmy has type 1 • Genetic • Diagnosed right after a viral illness	**Why Timmy's at high risk for type 2** • Low activity levels • High BMI (body mass index, a height-weight ratio; lower is healthier) • Family history • Poor diet • Extra weight located mostly around the middle
Prescription to reduce risk • No known way to prevent it	**Prescription to reduce risk** • Assess habits with the RealAge Healthy Kids Test and then improve overall lifestyle. • Slowly increase exercise/activity to 60 minutes a day (stamina and strength). • Adjust diet to replace most simple sugars (sweets, processed foods) with complex carbohydrates (fruits, veggies, whole grains).
Classic Symptoms • Significant weight loss • Frequent urination, especially at night • Increased thirst and appetite	**Early signs** • Excessive weight gain • Fatigue due to insulin resistance • Finding elevated blood sugar levels during routine physical exam
Daily routine • Strict diet to control blood sugar levels • Exercise (stamina and strength) • Monitor blood sugar level • Insulin injections	**Daily routine if he develops diabetes** • Strict diet to control blood sugar levels • Strict exercise program • Monitor blood sugar level • Possible medication regimen for the rest of his life
Risks of not managing condition • Blindness • Kidney failure • Diabetic shock • Heart disease and stroke • Circulatory issues/complications • Erectile dysfunction • Limb amputation • More susceptible to infectious diseases and complications	**Risks of not managing condition** • Blindness • Kidney failure • Diabetic shock • Heart disease and stroke • Circulatory issues/complications • Erectile dysfunction • Limb amputation • More susceptible to infectious diseases and complications

12 Questions That Will Help Prevent the Illnesses That Threaten Kids Most

While some diseases can't be prevented, many others can, including type 2 diabetes, heart disease, and high blood pressure. Jimmy needs to manage his type 1 diabetes, and Timmy needs to avoid developing type 2.

> *RealAge Projection:* Without good management, diabetes can dramatically undermine children's health, especially over time. If they fail to keep it under control as adults, their RealAge could be more like 40 when they're really in their mid-30s.

Remember, it's always the simple health habits that we let slip—small choices that turn into big problems down the road. In the past seven chapters we've covered several key areas; now let's step back and review. To get an overall picture of your child's health and how health-care providers fit in, ask yourself a few questions:

1. **Has your child had the recommended routine checkup(s) this year?**
Routine checkups are essential for kids, and I'm not saying that just because I'm a pediatrician. Checkups are when doctors often catch conditions such as the following—which, because the symptoms aren't always obvious, parents can easily miss.

- Vision problems
- Anemia
- Elevated lead levels

- Hypertension
- High cholesterol
- Kidney problems
- Hyperglycemia
- Hyperlipidemia
- Hearing problems

Regular checkups also ensure that any treatments for existing conditions are still working. Finally, regular checkups when kids are healthy help them feel at ease about going to the doctor when they're sick. A pediatrician isn't your only option, by the way; for other health-care choices, see page 63.

2. What does *regular* mean?

You and your doctor should decide how often your child needs to come in for checkups. I recommend the following schedule. It's more frequent than is currently recommended by the American Academy of Pediatrics, which establishes the minimum necessary to be sure a child is okay at the time of the visit. But my goal is to catch developmental problems early and *prevent* diseases down the road.

- Within one week of discharge from hospital
- Once a month for the first 6 months
- Every other month from 6 months to 12 months
- At 15 months, 18 months, 21 months, 2 years, 2.4 years, 2.8 years, 3 years, 3.5 years, 4 years, 4.5 years, and 5 years
- Yearly thereafter through age 18

What exactly happens at a routine visit? Checkups can involve some or all of these items, depending on the child's age:

- Head-to-toe exam—such as checking eyes, ears, nose, mouth, heart, organs, reflexes, muscle tone—as well as taking strength, and running urine and blood tests
- Measurements such as blood pressure, heart rate, and respiratory rate
- Body mass index (BMI) check to be sure height and weight are in healthy proportion to each other
- Vaccinations, if needed

The physical exam makes sure all your child's body systems are growing and working properly. Your pediatrician should also spend time asking about:

- **Eating,** such as appetite, dieting, obesity, and eating disorders
- **Exercise,** including how much, what kind, and how often
- **Hygiene,** including sleep habits, dental care, and hand-washing
- **Intellectual development,** including social skills and school performance
- **Emotional health and self-esteem,** including behavior, family dynamics, sibling rivalry, and peer relationships
- **Safety** at home, school, and while traveling, including use of child seats, seat belts, sunscreen, helmets

If your pediatrician isn't a big talker, jot down questions and concerns ahead of time—it can help make the most of your child's appointment. (If it's your first visit, flip to the end of this chapter for a worksheet on what the doctor needs to know about your child.)

3. **Has your child received all the recommended vaccinations?**

Immunizations and vaccinations are really the same thing. They help your child's body recognize and fight off infectious diseases. They also make it less likely that your protected child

Do Vaccinations Cause Autism?

One of the biggest fears about vaccinations is that some of them—particularly the MMR combination shot against measles, mumps, and rubella—might cause autism. Autism is a complex neurodevelopmental disorder that can range in severity. Symptoms include:

- impaired social interaction
- problems with verbal and nonverbal communication
- obsessive or repetitive routines
- restricted interests

Its cause is unclear, but it is generally accepted that autism is the result of an abnormality in the brain; however, researchers don't know why it occurs. In many cases the symptoms of autism are not apparent until 12 to 24 months.

The controversy about the MMR shot has arisen for a couple of reasons. First, the incidence of autism has increased since this particular vaccine was introduced. Second, signs of autism often appear around the time this vaccine is given. This has been studied and debated at length; however, the scientific evidence argues against the MMR connection.

While some suspected the MMR vaccine itself as a cause, others focused on a preservative called thimerosal. It guards against contamination, and contains minute amounts of mercury. It's the mercury that has been implicated as a potential cause of autism spectrum disorders (ASDs). And because thimerosal was used in many other vaccines as well, fears focused specifically around it have also spread.

So far, several major medical studies have found no causal link between the MMR vaccine and autism, or between thimerosal and autism, though research continues. Meanwhile, most childhood vaccines are now available in mercury-free formulations. If you have any concerns, ask your health-care provider to use only preservative-free vaccines.

will pass a disease on to someone else who isn't. Children must be given a complete series of shots to be fully protected; the immunization checklist on page 257 will help you keep track.

Vaccinations have helped save millions of lives around the world and have virtually eradicated many fatal diseases. Although there's a near-absence of many of these illnesses in the United States, they still exist—witness the mumps outbreak in 2006. It's important to be proactive with vaccinations to ensure these debilitating illnesses don't come back.

4. **Are you and your pediatrician routinely tracking your child's growth?**
Growth charts are used to see if children are developing at a normal rate. Measurements for infants include head circumference, length, and weight; for older children, height and weight, which are then compared with growth charts, including the body mass index (BMI), a weight/height ratio that indirectly gauges body fat composition.

You can calculate your child's BMI with the following formula:

Weight in pounds ÷ height (in inches ÷ height in inches × 703

So a 7-year-old child who weighs 50 pounds and is 4 feet tall (48 inches) has a BMI of 15.25:

$$50 \div 48 \div 48 \times 703 = 15.25$$

A BMI of 15.25 is likely to be a healthy number, and you can compare it to BMI charts for kids 2 to 20 years at the

Centers for Disease Control and Prevention (www.cdc.
gov).But it's a good idea to take your child's number to the
next routine checkup and discuss it with your pediatrician
because evaluating the BMI for children isn't that simple.
Children's body fat levels change frequently as they grow,
and differ for girls and boys.

That said, either slow or quick changes in height/weight
growth ratios could indicate issues with:

- Caloric intake
- Metabolism
- Gastrointestinal system
- Hormones (especially thy-
  roid growth hormone)
- A genetic disorder
- An eating disorder

> **Today's Child Is Heavier**
>
> In 1963, the average 10-year-old boy weighed about 74 pounds. In 2002, he weighed 85 pounds. That's a 14 percent increase! Height has gone up over time, too, but not enough to make up for the weight gain.

But only your child's doctor
can figure this out, because
growth patterns vary so much in kids.

5. **Are you tuned in to any worrisome weight gain?**
Obesity in children is rising. Today, 15 percent of children
are obese—meaning their weight is greater than the 95th
percentile for their age group. Obesity is specifically associated with thickening of the arterial wall, a classic precursor
to heart disease.

The subject of weight is touchy at any
age, but especially with children. Before you
start talking about weight to your child, you
must know exactly how to approach the topic
or you could make matters worse. For many

> Dieting in children can actually promote weight gain.

adolescents, dieting is not only ineffective, it may actually promote weight gain. One study in particular followed two groups of kids—some had frequently tried diets and some hadn't. After three years the dieters ended up gaining more weight than the nondieters.

If you realize that your child is gaining too much weight, don't try to tackle the situation by yourself. Talk to your pediatrician alone and then follow up with an appointment for your child. It may sound obvious, but your pediatrician will likely follow this approach:

- **Figure out the likely cause(s) of weight gain**: These include too little physical activity, diet changes, puberty, adolescence, stress, peer pressure, medications, and possibly medical conditions such as genetic syndromes and endocrinologic diseases (but only 5 percent or so of people have these).
- **Look at your child's eating habits, and the family's**: Consider not only breakfast, lunch, and dinner, but also snacking, desserts, and dining out (see Chapter 2).
- **Look at activity levels, too**: These include simply playing around, team and individual sports, walking to and from school, recess time, and family activities (see Chapter 3).
- **Evaluate mental and emotional health**: Gauge self-esteem, body image, confidence level, stress levels, depression, and willingness to make a change (see Chapter 6).

Once you've gone through the process together, you, your child, and your pediatrician can develop a safe, effective plan to help guide your child back to a healthy weight.

6. **Are you tuned in to any worrisome weight loss?**
Parents and pediatricians need to keep their antennae up for
clues that a child is trying to lose weight in an unhealthy way,
especially during adolescence. The desire to fit in or achieve
a "perfect" body type can lead adolescents down a dangerous
road.

Risky habits include avoiding meals; fasting; and using
laxative and diet pills, caffeine, and smoking as ways to
curb appetite. Hoarding food—stockpiling it in closets or
backpacks—could mean your child has developed a binge-
purge routine.

This kind of behavior is more common in girls than
boys, but it occurs in both.
Although body dissatisfaction
is often blamed on models and
superhero characters, it can
start much closer to home.
There's a strong link between
parents' attitudes about eating and body image and their
children's. In other words, if a
mom has a poor body image,
her child may too.

> **BMI and Cancer Risk**
>
> You might not believe it, but an over-
> weight child—one with a BMI in the
> 85–100th percentile for age and sex—
> has a far greater chance of getting can-
> cer later in life than an average-weight
> child. That's more reason than ever to
> keep kids active! Diet is also critical.
> Cutting down on red meat and salt has
> proven very effective when it comes to
> avoiding stomach and colon cancer.

So try to be the best role
model you can be. Don't put
yourself down. Don't try to
enforce a rigid diet. If you need to control your own weight,
do it in a safe, positive manner. *Show* your child that eating
more fruits and vegetables, and decreasing fats and sugars, is
healthier and more effective than the fad-diet-of-the-week.

In fact, just say no to diets. Sensible eating and exercise is the way to go. Remember, offer your kids nutritious

choices for meals and snacks, and help them learn how to balance food and physical activity. Refer back to Chapters 2 and 3 for specific strategies on encouraging lifelong eating and exercise patterns. In addition, the online tools in the box below will give you a better idea of exactly what and how much children need to eat at different ages.

7. **Do you keep your kids active?**
Without a doubt, regular physical activity is the best way to prevent weight gain and debilitating illnesses in the years ahead, such as osteoporosis, heart disease, cancer, and stroke. For the most part, young kids have no trouble getting their bodies jumping and hearts pumping. However, older children and adolescents who don't play sports often

---

Climbing the Pyramid

No doubt you're familiar with the food pyramid developed by the U.S. Department of Agriculture (USDA). Basically, it illustrates the recommended daily servings a person should eat from each of the basic food groups. The pyramid got a major update in April 2005, and now includes a version for children 6 to 11 years, and guidelines for younger and older children as well.

The pyramid is a good starting point, but keep in mind that it is only one guideline, not the end-all for healthful eating. For instance, the Harvard School of Public Health has created an admired alternative that emphasizes a foundation of daily exercise and weight control and offers somewhat more specific guidelines about certain foods.

I feel both programs are valuable and, if used together, let you create a personalized program for your child.

The USDA's version is at: mypyramid.gov.

The Harvard alternative is at: www.hsph.harvard.edu/nutritionsource/pyramids.html.

fall short on physical activity. In fact, a recent study found that one in three teens is too out of shape to complete a simple treadmill fitness test. That's not good. No child should be a fitness failure.

If team sports aren't up a kid's alley, suggest more individual activities—dance classes, martial arts, horseback riding, pole vaulting, yoga, whatever. Pretty much any activity that gets them up and moving is fine. They just have to like it enough to do it on most days.

Kids who find activities they enjoy regularly cope better with stress at school or home; they worry less and laugh more; and their bodies work better, thanks to stronger muscles, bones, and joints. Plus, staying fit helps kids feel good about themselves and builds self-confidence, which can help them avoid dangers such as drug and alcohol use now and later.

8. How's the household hygiene?

What fun is a checkup without some talk of germs? Something as simple as getting kids into the habit of washing their hands frequently works wonders at reducing colds and infectious illnesses. Check to make sure they're scrubbing both the backs and fronts of hands, between fingers, under the nails—and that they spend at least fifteen seconds doing it. That's about the amount of time it takes to sing "Happy Birthday" or chant the alphabet.

Still, don't turn your child into a germaphobe. Go easy on the antibacterial products. Flip back to Chapter 4 for a rundown of which germs you and your child really need to watch out for—and which ones are actually good for you.

9. **Are you comfortable with their social and intellectual development?**

It's natural for parents to wonder if their kids are developing normally. That's another reason for routine checkups. Here are examples of questions your pediatrician might ask to gauge how a child has progressed intellectually and behaviorally since the last visit:

- At 18 months: Has your child started to speak? Imitate your actions? Are tantrums a concern?
- At 2 years: Is your child sleeping through the night? Eating with a fork or spoon? Running? Turning pages in a book?
- At 6 years: Does your kid like reading? Wet the bed at night?
- At 10 years: Is your child struggling at school? Able to use the computer?

To check physical development, your pediatrician may ask a 4-year-old to hop on one foot, do jumping jacks, manipulate small objects, and do some drawings.

Social and emotional milestones are often harder to pinpoint, but they're just as important. Basically, the pediatrician wants to assess whether a child is developing a healthy sense of self and has age-appropriate social skills. In young kids, this can be seen in whether they express a wide range of emotions and how well they relate to the people around them. As children get older, pediatricians want to know how they function in more structured groups. Do they handle sharing and taking turns? Do they get along with siblings? Do they have good friends? Are they cooperative? Do they respond to the feelings of others?

Many parents don't voice concerns about emotional

issues unless their pediatrician initiates the conversation. But don't hesitate to get things out in the open. The earlier social-emotional problems are recognized, the better the outcome is likely to be. (See Chapter 6 for more about self-esteem and emotional health.)

Finally, remember that there are no firm rules when it comes to development. You must always keep *your* child's age, stage, temperament, and learning style in mind.

10. **Do your kids—and you—put safety first?**
Most childhood injuries are from accidents. And while accidents aren't always preventable, a seat belt or bike helmet can prevent disabling injuries, including paralysis, amnesia, slurred speech, depression, anxiety, and loss of motor skills.

Parents' perceptions of their children's safety habits aren't always correct. They may think their kids wear helmets or sunscreen when actually they don't. Chapter 7 focuses on how to instill habits that will help prevent accidents and injuries.

11. **What if your child has a chronic health problem?**
More than 15 percent of children in the United States have chronic medical conditions. Teaching kids how to manage a specific condition on a day-to-day basis can mean the difference between a long, happy life and a short, bedridden one. It may sound harsh, but it's true. The better your family understands the condition and its treatment, the better you'll be able to help your child control it. Keep up to date on the research. (RealAge.com has an expert-driven search engine that's very useful for finding the latest medical studies.)

12. Have you instilled the "4 Is" in yourself?

Remember those four steps we talked about in Chapter 1—*identify*, *inform*, *instruct*, and *instill*? Regular checkups help you focus on the first three. But you're totally in charge of the last "I": instilling healthy habits. Children depend on parents for guidance and support, and need reminders about rules and limits. Reinforcing healthy habits along the way will teach kids moderation, discretion, consistency, and self-discipline.

Over time, kids will develop their own sense of self-control, and maintain healthy habits for themselves. That will help them enjoy good health for years to come.

RealAge Projection: Learning to be proactive about health issues will benefit kids indefinitely. If they keep it up into adulthood, at 50 they could look and feel closer to 38!

Immunization Checklist for Your Child

Use this checklist to keep track of the vaccinations your child receives. Simply fill in the date of each shot. Always check with your child's physician, pediatrician, or health-care provider for the most current information or if you have any questions or concerns.

Child's name: _____

Birth date: _____

Vaccine	Protects Against	Dates Given	Notes
HepB	Hepatitis B—a virus that causes chronic liver disease or cirrhosis	1. _____ (Birth–2 mos) 2. _____ (1–4 mos) 3. _____ (6–18 mos)	
DTaP	• Diphtheria, an infectious disease that may affect nose, throat, and skin • Tetanus (lockjaw), an infectious disease of the central nervous system • Pertussis (whooping cough), a contagious disease that causes violent coughing spasms	1. _____ (2 mos) 2. _____ (4 mos) 3. _____ (6 mos) 4. _____ (15–18 mos) 5. _____ (4–6 years) 6. _____ (11–12 years) Every 10 years thereafter	
Hib (Haemophilus influenzae type b)	Bacterial meningitis (an infection of the brain/spinal cord), pneumonia, and blood infections	1. _____ (2 mos) 2. _____ (4 mos) 3. _____ (6 mos) 4. _____ (12–15 mos)	

Vaccine	Protects Against	Dates Given	Notes
MCV4	Meningoccal meningitis; a form of bacterial meningitis that's more prevalent in adolescents	Usually given at age 11–12; essential before going to sleep-away camps or living in dorms	
IPV (Inactivated Poliovirus)	Polio, an infectious disease that affects the whole body, including muscles and nerves	1. _____ (2 mos) 2. _____ (4 mos) 3. _____ (6-18 mos) 4. _____ (4–6 years)	Final dose must be given after 4th birth-day
PCV	Pneumococcal disease, common cause of bacterial meningitis, and bacterial pneumonia	1. _____ (2 mos) 2. _____ (4 mos) 3. _____ (6 mos) 4. _____ (12–15 mos)	
MMR	• Measles, a highly contagious illness marked by tiny red spots • Mumps, a contagious disease that causes painful swelling of the salivary glands • Rubella (German measles), a contagious disease marked by a rash	1. _____ (12–15 mos) 2. _____ (4–6 years)	First dose must be given on or after 1st birthday
Varicella	Chickenpox, a classic childhood disease characterized by itchy, fluid-filled blisters	1. _____ (12–18 mos)	

Vaccine	Protects Against	Dates Given	Notes
HepA	Hepatitis A virus, a viral disease that causes inflammation of the liver; often from contaminated water or food, or poor hygiene	1. _____ (12+ mos) 2. _____ (18+ mos)	Second dose is given no sooner than 6 months after the first
Vaccine	**Protects Against**	**Dates Given**	**Notes**
Influenza	The flu, a contagious respiratory illness	Yearly between 6 months and 5 years: optional but frequently recommended after age 5	Given yearly
HPV	Human papillomavirus, a sexually transmitted disease that causes genital warts and cervical cancer	1. _____ (9–12 years) 2. _____ (2 mos after 1st dose) 3. _____ (6 mos after 1st dose)	
Rotavirus	Highly contagious gastrointestinal infection; major cause of vomiting and diarrhea in young children	1. _____ (2 mos) 2. _____ (4 mos) 3. _____ (6 mos)	A series of 3 doses, given orally over 6 months

Based on the Centers for Disease Control and Prevention recommendations as of December 1, 2005.

What Your Pediatrician Needs to Know About Your Child

To prepare for a first visit, here's a basic list of all the things that a new doctor doesn't yet know about your kid, and needs to.

☐ Full name _____

☐ Birth date _____

☐ Current height and weight _____ ft. _____ in. _____ lbs.

☐ Date of last checkup _____

☐ Current immunizations _____

    HepB 1. _____ 2. _____ 3. _____

    DTaP 1. _____ 2. _____ 3. _____ 4. _____ 5. _____ 6. _____

    Hib 1. _____ 2. _____ 3. _____ 4. _____

    MCV4 _____

    IPV 1. _____ 2. _____ 3. _____ 4. _____

    Varicella _____

    PCV 1. _____ 2. _____ 3. _____ 4. _____

    MMR 1. _____ 2. _____

    HepA 1. _____ 2. _____

    HPV 1. _____ 2. _____ 3. _____

    Rotovirus 1. _____ 2. _____ 3. _____

☐ Immunization reactions, if any _____

_____

☐ General health history _____

_____

_____

☐ Any current illnesses and symptoms _____

_____

_____

☐ Any chronic illnesses/conditions (e.g., asthma, epilepsy) _____

_____

_____

☐ Treatments for any of the above _____

_____

_____

☐ Any allergies (e.g., food, medications, insects) _____

_____

_____

☐ Any medications (include doses and schedule) _____

_____

_____

☐ Sleep/nap routine _____

_____

_____

☐ Vitamins, supplements (include dose and schedule) _____

_____

_____

☐ Any hospitalizations

    Date _____ Reason _____

    Date _____ Reason _____

    Date _____ Reason _____

☐ Any surgeries

    Date _____ Reason _____

    Date _____ Reason _____

    Date _____ Reason _____

☐ Any fears or phobias _____

_____

☐ Favorite foods _____

_____

☐ Hobbies, sports, extracurricular activities _____

_____

☐ Any siblings _____

_____

_____

☐ Any pets _____

_____

☐ Family or social circumstances that may affect your child _____

_____

_____

How to Select the Right Health-Care Provider for Your Child

First, you need to decide what kind of practitioner will suit your family best. The three most common providers of children's medical care are:

☐ Pediatricians—physicians who specialize in the care of kids from birth through young adulthood

☐ Family physicians/practitioners—doctors who provide health care for all members of the family

☐ Pediatric nurse practitioners—RNs with advanced training who provide some primary care for kids and can do many basic tasks performed by physicians as well

Once you've decided what type appeals to you the most, ask around for some recommendations, narrow your list, call their offices, and ask a few questions:

☐ What are your office hours? *(Are they convenient for your schedule?)*

☐ How many doctors are in the practice? *(More may be better; you'll have backups in case your doctor is unavailable.)*

☐ Which hospital are you affiliated with? *(How does it compare with others in your area? Is it convenient?)*

☐ What types of insurance plans do you participate in? *(It's best to double-check!)*

Finally, meet the candidates who seem to fit you best face-to-face. Many parents do this even before their first baby is born. If you already have kids, bring them along; their reaction is important, too. Consider the following during your meeting:

☐ Does the doctor make you and your children feel comfortable?

☐ Does the doctor talk directly to the kids?

☐ Does the doctor explain things well? In language children can understand?

☐ Does the doctor listen to questions and concerns, or seem rushed for time?

☐ Do you share similar philosophies on child-rearing issues (such as breastfeeding, circumcision, sleep training, diet, exercise)?

Many of the charts and checklists in this chapter can be printed out at
www.RealAge.com/parenting

Teaching a Child How to Cope with a Chronic Condition

The following conditions are listed alphabetically, not by frequency, so it's easy to skip to the ones that interest you. Keep in mind that this list is for quick reference; only a doctor can diagnose and treat illness.

ALLERGIES AND SINUS PROBLEMS

Description: An exaggerated immune response to a variety of substances, from food to pets, mold to plants. Symptoms can include sinus pain and inflammation, itchy eyes, nasal congestion, rashes, hives, scratchy throat, and difficulty breathing.

Frequency: Of all chronic conditions affecting kids, allergies are among the most common. The good news is that children sometimes outgrow allergies.

Causes: Most kids with allergies inherit a tendency to have them, and kids with eczema are more likely to have allergies.

Treatment: A doctor should assess what's triggering allergic reactions, asking about food, environment, what's different now that didn't exist before the reaction, and much more. You and your child need to watch these potential triggers and make a note if a reaction occurs. If you can't figure it out this way, a blood test known as RAST or a scratch skin test might identify the cause.

Once the cause is known, the goal is to avoid it. When that's not possible—it's hard to avoid grass or dust, for instance—over-the-counter (OTC) or prescription antihistamines can prevent or calm down the reaction. Many short-acting OTC antihistamines may cause drowsiness; however, formulas such as Claritin and Alavert are nonsedating and long-acting, and no longer require a prescription. If they aren't sufficient, there are prescription options, including nasal steroids and eye drops.

Severe allergies may require a series of allergy shots—given when the cause can't be avoided and the symptoms are unbearable. For allergic emergencies—such as severe reactions to bee stings—get a prescription for an EpiPen, which auto-injects epinephrine via a lightweight "pen." Keep it handy at all times.

Untreated allergies can lead to long-term health complications, such as chronic ear or sinus problems. Sneezing, wheezing, dripping, and tearing can keep a child out of physical activities—especially outdoors—increasing the risk of weight and cardiovascular problems.

Learn more:

The Food Allergy and Anaphylaxis Network
        www.foodallergy.org
The American Academy of Allergy, Asthma, and
        Immunology
        www.aaaai.org

ANEMIA/IRON DEFICIENCY

Description: A lack of iron—and when the body lacks iron, it cannot make enough hemoglobin, the substance in red blood cells that carries oxygen to the body and brain.

Frequency: Infants, toddlers, preschoolers, and adolescent girls are most at risk. In one study, about 7 percent of 1- to 2-year-olds showed signs of deficiency; in adolescent girls, the incidence may be 9 to 16 percent. Vegetarians are also at a greater risk.

Cause: In general, a lack of iron-rich foods and menstruation are the most common causes.

Treatment: Iron supplements will help boost iron levels and build up iron stores in the body. Good diet sources include leafy green vegetables, red meat, dark poultry, eggs, and dried fruits. Newborns get iron from one of the best sources: breast milk. If not breastfeeding, use iron-enriched formula. Getting enough vitamin C also aids the body's absorption of iron.

Untreated iron deficiency can permanently impact brain development, making it hard for children to learn. Iron-deficient kids also may not gain enough weight or grow properly, tire easily, have digestion problems, and be prone to infections and illness. Iron deficiency also increases lead absorption, so the risk of lead poisoning is higher.

ASTHMA

Description: A respiratory disease that constricts the small vessels in the lungs, making breathing difficult and sometimes impossible.

Frequency: Rates of asthma have increased around the world. Currently, an estimated 4 million children under 18 have had an asthma attack in the past twelve months, and many others have undiagnosed asthma.

Causes: There is evidence that many factors, genetic and environmental, play a part. Like allergies, asthma tends to run in families.

Treatment: Although asthma cannot be cured, it can almost always be controlled. The number one thing *you* can do for your child's asthma is DON'T SMOKE. This is vital for all children, but it's doubly so for asthmatic ones.

As with allergies, identifying what triggers asthma attacks is key to managing the condition. Once you've identified the triggers, you can both work to avoid them. Bronchodilaters (inhalers) and anti-inflammatory medications also are often prescribed.

If asthma is not controlled, it can cause long-term sleep problems due to breathing restriction, a weakened immune system, reduced cognitive ability, learning difficulties, and, over time, loss of lung function.

Learn more:

American Academy of Allergy, Asthma, and Immunology
    www.aaaai.org

ATTENTION DEFICIT HYPERACTIVITY DISORDER (ADHD)

Description: Condition marked by short attention span, over-activity, and impulsive behavior.

Frequency: Between 3 and 5 percent of school-aged children have some level of ADHD (sometimes known as ADD); it's more prevalent in boys than girls.

Causes: As far as we know, children are born with this genetic condition.

Treatment: Usually managed with a combination of behavioral therapy and medication. When properly managed, children may learn to use their excess energy to their advantage, while also learning to minimize less productive tendencies. A healthy diet, high-quality sleep, and limited distractions can help. (See Chapter 5 for more information on ADHD.) Failing to spot and treat ADHD in childhood may damage overall health and well-being into adulthood. It ups the lifetime risk of school failure, depression, behavioral disorders, work and relationship problems, and substance abuse.

Learn more:

CHADD: Children and Adults with Attention-Deficit/
    Hyperactivity Disorder
    www.chadd.org
Learning Disabilities Online: ADD/ADHD,
    www.ldonline.org

Autism Spectrum Disorders (ASDs)

Description: A complex neurodevelopmental disorder, appearing during the first three years of life and affecting people to varying degrees. Symptoms include poor social interaction, problems with verbal and nonverbal communication, obsessive or repetitive routines, and restricted interests.

Frequency: About 1 in 166 children is affected by autism; it is four times more common in boys than girls.

Causes: The cause is unknown, but genetic and environmental factors may play a role. It results from abnormal development of certain parts of the brain.

Treatment: Treatment can be as complex as the disease itself, and depends on the severity and the child. Early, intensive education and therapy can help children develop and learn skills that help them communicate, interact, play, learn, and take care of themselves. This also can help with the difficult symptoms of an ASD in a child. Certain medications also are sometimes used to reduce symptoms such as anxiety, anger, and repetitive behaviors.

Learn more:

Centers for Disease Control and Prevention: National Center on Birth Defects and Developmental Disabilities: Autism

www.cdc.gov/ncbdd/ddautism.htm

Autism Speaks

www.autismspeaks.org

BLINDNESS

Description: To be legally blind, a child must have vision worse than 20/200, or have a field of vision less than 20 degrees in the better eye.

Frequency in children: Approximately 13.5 million children between birth and age 17 suffer partial or complete blindness.

Causes: In children, vision impairment may be due to birth defects. Optic nerve damage, injury of the eye(s), and trauma to the part of the brain that controls vision may also result in blindness. So can bilateral congenital cataracts, which may cloud the lenses so that light can't pass through.

Treatment: Ongoing instruction from specially trained teachers and therapists can provide the communication, academic, social, and other skills that visually impaired children need to thrive. If not properly managed, vision impairments can lead to social isolation, depression, and injury.

Learn more:

Lighthouse International

www.lighthouse.org

Prevent Blindness America

www.preventblindness.org/children

CANCER

Description: Malignant growth or tumor caused by abnormal cells that can invade and damage healthy tissue.

Frequency: Childhood cancer is relatively rare. It affects about 14 of every 100,000 children in the United States each year. The most common childhood cancers are bone marrow (leukemia), lymphatic (lymphoma), and brain.

Causes: It's a great mystery. Many contributors are suspected, including genetic predisposition, exposure to certain toxins or chemicals, prolonged exposure to the sun's UV rays, and radiation.

Treatment: Whatever the cause, treatments exist, research progresses—and the mortality rate has dropped. Surgery, chemotherapy, and radiation, alone or in combination, are the most effective treatments. Medical centers specializing in childhood cancer have psychologists, social workers, child experts, nutritionists, physical therapists, and educators who support and educate the entire family. This kind of network guiding kids and families through the process makes it much more manageable.

Learn more:

National Cancer Institute

www.cancer.gov/cancertopics/types/childhoodcancers

CYSTIC FIBROSIS (CF)

Description: Hereditary metabolic disorder characterized by abnormal production of thick mucus. Primarily affects the pancreas and respiratory system and results in chronic infection.

Frequency: An estimated 2,500 babies are born with CF each year and more than 30,000 children and young adults in the United States have it.

Cause: It's a metabolic disorder that's passed from parent to child. It's seen mostly in Caucasians of Central and Northern European descent, but affects every race.

Treatment: Preventing infection with antibiotics, reducing the amount and thickness of secretions with mucus-thinning drugs, and improving air flow with bronchodilators may slow lung deterioration in some children. Treatment with ibuprofen may also help. Physical methods that work to maintain lung function and avoid complications include the airway clearance technique (ACT) and daily postural drainage and chest percussion (PD&P), a form of physical therapy.

Adequate calories and good nutrition are critical, and pancreatic enzyme replacement is often needed to help digestion. In the most extreme cases, a lung transplant may be required. Without proper management, a child with CF will suffer chronic respiratory and digestive infections, and early mortality.

Learn more:

Cystic Fibrosis Foundation
    www.ccf.org

DEPRESSION

Description: A condition characterized by ongoing feelings of overwhelming sadness and despair.

Frequency: Incidence increases with age. Approximately 1 to 3 percent of children under 10 are diagnosed as depressed. In teens, the rate rises to 3 to 6 percent. The numbers are higher if other family members are depressed.

Cause: Although the exact cause of clinical depression is not fully understood, it appears to be a combination of several factors—biological, genetic, environmental, and/or childhood events.

Treatment: The earlier depression is recognized and treated, the better the prognosis. With therapy, medication, or both, kids can go on to lead happy, healthy lives. Talk therapy may work on its own; however, there are also many antidepressant medications that are effective. But because some have potentially risky side effects, close monitoring by a physician is absolutely essential.

Left untreated, depression can interfere greatly with the development, well-being, and future health and happiness of your child. It can lead to eating or sleep disorders, obesity, and substance abuse in adulthood, and suicide, which is the second leading cause of adolescent death after motor vehicle accidents.

Learn more:

Parentsmedguide.org

The Use of Medication in Treating Childhood and
Adolescent Depression

www.parentsmedguide.org

DIABETES: TYPE 1 AND TYPE 2

Description: Insufficient insulin production leading to poor
metabolism of glucose. Type 1, or insulin-dependent diabetes, is typically first seen in childhood and is not
preventable. Type 2, insulin-resistant diabetes, is more common in adults but it's rapidly increasing in children. It is
strongly tied to being overweight and inactive, so a change
in lifestyle—weight, diet, exercise—is the most effective
way to both prevent and manage it.

Frequency: About 1 of every 400 to 500 kids has diabetes.
While roughly 13,000 children are diagnosed with type 1
each year, the Centers for Disease Control and Prevention
believe that new cases of type 2 account for 8 to 43 percent
of all diabetes diagnosed.

Cause: Genes play a role but a minor one in type 2. Lifestyle
factors, such as poor diet and lack of physical activity,
account for 90 to 95 percent of type 2 diabetes.

Treatment: Children with diabetes must be taught how to recognize and control low blood sugar. Exercise and diet are
vital for both types in order to maintain blood sugar levels
and normal weight. In addition, type 1 requires injecting
insulin under the skin one to four times a day and type
2 may require similar injections. If insulin injections are
necessary, kids must learn how to do it themselves.

If either type 1 or 2 diabetes is not well controlled, it
can gradually lead to heart attacks, strokes, blindness, kid-

ney failure, gum disease, blood vessel disease, nerve damage, amputation, and impotence in men.

Learn more:

American Diabetes Association

www.diabetes.org/for-parents-and-kids.jsp

DOWN SYNDROME

Description: An inherited chromosomal disorder, diagnosed before or at birth. Results in some degree of mental retardation.

Frequency: Occurs in 1 out of every 660 births and is diagnosed before or at birth. Symptoms vary widely.

Cause: Children with Down syndrome inherit an extra copy of the twenty-first chromosome, which causes developmental delays, and often leads to mental retardation. No one knows for sure why Down occurs. Women over age 35 have a significantly higher risk of having a child with the condition.

Treatment: There is no specific medical treatment, but there are many educational and support systems for families with Down syndrome children, including the National Down Syndrome Congress.

Children with Down syndrome are more susceptible to other health issues such as ear and sinus infections, constipation, joint problems, heart trouble, and vision and hearing problems.

Learn more:

National Down Syndrome Society

www.ndss.org

ECZEMA

Description: Inflammation of the skin. Characterized by itching and scaling; may lead to lesions that crust over. Can be acute or chronic.

Frequency: Eczema usually first appears in infancy and about 15 to 20 percent of school-age kids have it. Happily, most kids eventually outgrow it.

Cause: The causes aren't completely clear but heredity plays a role, so if one family member has eczema, it's more likely that a child will, too.

Treatment: Management includes identifying and avoiding whatever aggravates the child's skin, which can be anything from certain foods to lanolin, a derivative of wool. Ointments and creams soothe irritation, and anti-itch medications are sometimes prescribed as well. Often, steroid-based creams are needed; however, some new nonsteroidal creams are now available with a prescription. Moisturize skin daily. Try to keep kids from scratching and keep nails short to avoid skin infections.

Learn more:

National Eczema Society

> www.eczema.org

GASTROESOPHAGEAL REFLUX DISEASE (GERD)

Description: GERD results from stomach acid backing up into the esophagus, causing a burning sensation. It is common in infants, especially premature babies. It's what causes them to spit up breast milk or formula during the first year of life.

Frequency: Although it usually stops around age 1, an estimated 3 to 5 percent of kids in the United States have reflux.

Cause: Genetics seems to be a key factor, but allergies, dietary intolerances, and other digestive disorders may play a role. Children with asthma, cystic fibrosis, and muscular or neurological problems and conditions such as Down syndrome are more likely to have GERD.

Treatment: Treatment depends on symptoms and age. If your child is uncomfortable, has difficulty sleeping or eating, or isn't growing, a doctor may try OTC or prescription antacids. Other treatments include eating smaller meals, not lying down right after eating, and sleeping with a bit of elevation to the head. GERD can often be managed by avoiding chocolate, caffeine, spicy foods, peppermint, carbonated drinks, and foods high in fat or acid.

Learn more:

National Digestive Diseases Information Clearinghouse
digestive.niddk.nih.gov/ddiseases/pubs/gerd/

HEARING IMPAIRMENTS

Description: Complete or partial loss of hearing ability.

Frequency: Roughly 3 out of every 1,000 babies are born with significant hearing loss, and many more are born with milder hearing loss. Overall, 3 to 5 percent of children 18 and under have some hearing loss.

Cause: Hearing loss is one of the most common birth defects. It also can come from infection or trauma, like a tear in the eardrum or a skull fracture. Temporary hearing loss might even come from a buildup of wax in the ear canal, something lodged in the ear, or an allergy or infection.

Treatment: Proper training, instruction, and treatment programs can make a huge difference by teaching kids how to cope, make productive use of residual hearing, improve communications, and use listening devices effectively. Hearing aids can help, as can surgical procedures, such as cochlear implants.

If not well managed, hearing loss can affect speech and language development, academic capabilities, self-image, and social/emotional development.

Learn more:

National Institute on Deafness and Other
Communication Disorders
www.nidcd.nih.gov

HIGH BLOOD PRESSURE/HYPERTENSION

Description: Elevation of blood pressure beyond the normal range for age and size.

Frequency: A recent study funded by the National Heart, Lung, and Blood Institute showed that blood pressure levels for children and teenagers have risen dramatically since 1988. But the range of normal varies widely in kids, depending on age, size, and gender, so what's acceptable in one child will raise a red flag in another. Your pediatrician is the best person to determine if your child's blood pressure is above normal.

Cause: Certain heart, lung, and kidney conditions can cause high blood pressure in children. But more and more childhood hypertension is due to obesity and a sedentary lifestyle.

Treatment: Healthy lifestyle adjustments can reduce high blood pressure caused by excess weight and lack of exercise. Eating a healthy/low-sodium diet (chapter 2), getting more exercise (Chapter 3), and managing daily stress (Chapter 6) can work wonders.

JUVENILE RHEUMATOID ARTHRITIS (JRA)

Description: A chronic autoimmune disease affecting the joints. Inflammation causes painful swelling and tenderness.

Frequency: Between 30,000 and 50,000 children in the United States are affected by this joint disease.

Cause: It's unknown.

Treatment: In about half the cases, juvenile rheumatoid arthritis subsides with time. Overall, children with JRA do very well with treatment to reduce joint pain, prevent joint damage, and maintain physical function.

JRA is often combatted with a combination of medications, physical therapy, and exercise. Anti-inflammatory agents like ibuprofen are sometimes prescribed, as well as some steroids. Glucosamine and chondroitin sulfate supplements sometimes help. Physical therapy helps kids build joint-supportive muscle and regain full range of motion in affected areas.

Learn more:

National Institute of Arthritis and Musculoskeletal and Skin Diseases: Questions and Answers About Juvenile Rheumatoid Arthritis
www.niams.nih.gov/hi/topics/juvenile_arthritis /juvarthr.htm

SICKLE CELL ANEMIA

Description: An inherited type of anemia due to abnormally shaped hemoglobin; causes joint pain, jaundice, lower limb ulcers, and fever, and can shorten life span.

Frequency: In the United States, it is most prevalent among children of African Americans (approximately 1 in 500) and those of Hispanic descent (approximately 1 in 1,200).

Cause: The disorder produces abnormal hemoglobin, a protein that enables red blood cells to carry oxygen to all parts of the body. This leads to early death of some red blood cells, causing anemia. Anemia can lead to shortness of breath, fatigue, and delayed growth and development. A rapid breakdown of red blood cells may also yellow the eyes and skin (jaundice). Symptoms vary from person to person; some cases are mild, while others require hospitalization.

Treatment: Although there is no known cure, it's quite possible for a child to maintain a good quality of life. However, ongoing treatment is needed for this condition. Folic acid helps a lot because it aids in producing new red blood cells. An anticancer drug, Hydroxyurea, reduces painful crises and treats acute chest syndrome. Vaccines and antibiotics help stave off infections. Red blood cell transfusions may be given. Bone marrow transplants are called for on occasion.

The most critical time to start treating sickle cell is in the first few years of life. That's when fragile systems are most vulnerable to damage and infection. Lack of proper treatment can cause pain, gallstones, and increased risk of infections.

Learn more:

Medline Plus—Sickle Cell Anemia
      www.nim.nih.org/medlineplus/sicklecellanemia.html
American Sickle Cell Anemia Association
      www.ascaa.org

SLEEP DISORDERS

Description: Sleep disorders encompass many different problems, but can be boiled down to four categories:

- Difficulty falling asleep
- Difficulty staying asleep
- Not being able to stay awake during the day
- Not being able to keep to a regular sleep schedule

Frequency: Sleep problems are common but often overlooked in children.

Cause: Many childhood sleep problems are related to poor sleep habits or an inconsistent bedtime routine, but sometimes stress, worry, or anxiety causes insomnia. Persistent sleep problems may also be symptoms of emotional difficulties.

Treatment: Developing consistent bedtime routines helps minimize most common problems. Sleep clinics can help with more serious disorders, and teach children techniques for relaxation.

Making sure children get enough sleep is a basic component of good health. Lack of rest throws the body out of balance and disrupts sensitive systems, affecting mood, school performance, and a host of other things.

Learn more:

American Academy of Child and Adolescent Psychiatry
    www.aacap.org (search under "sleep")

URINARY TRACT INFECTIONS (UTIs)

Description: Infection, inflammation, and irritation of the bladder caused by bacteria traveling up the urethra. Also known as cystitis.

Frequency: Incidence seems to be highest in kids under age 2, with most infections occurring in the first year. The rate isn't very high when you look at the overall population—somewhere around 2 percent—but it can be painful and requires treatment to prevent a more serious kidney infection.

Cause: Some children are born with urinary reflux, a condition where urine flows back from the bladder to the kidneys, causing frequent infections in the urinary tract. But usually the urethra is irritated by other matter—bubble bath, perfumed soaps, fecal soiling, wet bathing suits—which makes an infection more likely.

Treatment: UTIs are generally treated with antibiotics. Urinary reflux is often treated with preventive, ongoing antibiotics until the child outgrows the condition. However, sometimes surgery is needed to correct the problem. (See Chapter 4 for more) If undetected, urologic diseases, such as urinary reflux, can do serious damage and lead to scarring of the kidneys.

Learn more:

National Kidney and Urologic Diseases Information
Clearinghouse
www.kidney.niddk.nik.gov
(search under "UTI children")

LIVE IT UP
Looking Forward to a Healthy Future

I was only three weeks from finishing up this book when I was invited to a child's birthday party—one I couldn't miss. Audrey was a childhood friend of my sister's, and this was her first baby's first birthday. I had known Audrey for years—she practically lived at our house growing up—and pretty much the whole family didn't think she'd ever choose to have kids. But here she was, the proud mom of a healthy 1-year-old boy.

My boys (my two sons and hubby) planned a guys-only day of hiking and bird spotting at the park; I brought my daughter, Emily, with me for the drive out to the country.

I gave my two sisters a sisters-only "look" when we arrived. Audrey was transformed. The quiet and serious girl I always remembered now had a circle of kids around her giggling uncontrollably as she and Tookie the Clown made crazy balloon animals—motherhood had brought out her silly side. In addition to the clown, she had hired a neighborhood teen to do arts and crafts with the kids, and my daughter Emily quickly spotted a tube of red glitter and plopped down at the table to create a sparkly masterpiece.

After introductions, I settled into a floral upholstered chair and took in the bustling room. Everyone had at least one child. Some were single parents, some married. I knew at least one who shared custody with her ex. A couple of Audrey's friends were pregnant, and everyone—including me—was offering the two women tips and pointers on parenting that they'd learned while raising their kids. We were so excited for the fun and challenging years that lay ahead for these expectant moms.

I thought I had to write this book to share everything I had learned as a pediatrician about being the best parent possible, about helping children develop healthy habits and be as happy, healthy, and successful as possible in the years ahead. But an interesting thing happened in the process. Even though I knew I had a knack for interpreting parent-child relationships in my office, after poring through all the research for the book, I realized that I had gained new perspective on the family dynamic. More than ever, I realized that there wasn't a "one size fits all" healthy lifestyle that worked for every family.

A woman to my right struck up a conversation starting with, "So I hear you're a pediatrician?" I smiled and asked about her kids (two girls, 10 and 6), and their interests (reading and gymnastics), and waited as she inevitably started in with child health questions. Not that I mind listening—it's my love, my pride to be a pediatrician—I just have always felt a little awkward giving specific advice without knowing a child first. I guess that's where my new perspective fits in; I found myself aching to tell her everything I learned while researching this book. I wanted to explain how it's her child's everyday routines and rituals that will really make good health stick. At the same time, I knew I couldn't sum it all up in a couple of sentences, so I bit my lip.

She had been talking about what a relief it would be when her kids were old enough to stay home for short bits of time alone, when she wouldn't have to be so diligent about their teeth brushing or fitness or not getting hurt. I felt so conflicted. Yes, 13-year-olds are more responsible for their own safety and well-being than 6-year-olds. But still, parents need to be at least as diligent during those early teen years as they are with toddlers. As teens begin to find their own way, they need guidance and inspiration to choose the healthiest path more than ever.

In fact, a recent study has shown that active kids often become inactive teens when the choice is entirely left up to them, and inactive teens then become inactive adults—and we know where that gets us. Just goes to show that good habits can slide at any time. Not that they can't be reversed . . .

At that moment, Emily ran up and motioned for me to lean down so she could tell me a secret. I smiled and nodded, and she ran back to the art table.

"You must be a Supermom," the woman to my right said, "with everything you know."

"Oh, no, far from it," I responded.

Because, let's be honest, knowing what to do and actually doing it are two very different things. Instead, I take what I know and try to make it work for my family.

In fact, I find that being imperfect is the best way to be. I strive to be the best role model for my kids, but I also let myself slip now and then. I try to provide the most nutritious foods, but we all get cravings. My husband and I always tell our kids, "McDonald's is okay once in a while." And our kids will occasionally ask, "Is it once in a while yet?" Code words for moderating indulgences. And when we do indulge, my daughter will say, "If I eat this now, then later I'll eat a healthy snack [like a banana or yogurt] to keep me growing strong." I love it.

Yes, guidance and inspiration all the way . . . but we're also human, and kids need to know it's okay not to be perfect. Rather than worrying about every indulgence, I focus on helping my kids see how making healthy choices fits in the big picture of their lives. I want to empower them to choose wisely for themselves.

So I wanted to tell the woman at the party, "Ohhh, you have to read my book, and then just do the best you can—that will be good enough. In fact, it'll be just fine." As a parent, you know way more than you think you do. Love goes a long way, after all.

BOOT UP
Online Tools, Resources, and Inspiration to Help Your Family Grow Healthier

▶ **Start with:**

RealAge Parenting

You can take the free RealAge Healthy Kids Test online here and not only will the computer calculate your score, but it will also generate an in-depth, activity-packed plan tailored to your child's needs. Plus you can sign up for free weekly tips from health experts, read and post messages on discussion boards, print out coloring pages, and download many of the charts and checklists in this book.

www.RealAge.com/parenting

RealAge

Parents with the healthiest lifestyles tend to raise the healthiest children, who, in turn, grow up to be healthier adults. Take stock of your own daily habits, parents, and give your lifestyle a healthy boost by taking the RealAge Test. You'll learn your

RealAge, or biological age, and get a personalized Age Reduction Plan just for you.

www.RealAge.com

▶ **For general health information about children, check out:**

American Academy of Family Physicians (AAFP)
Explore a wealth of practical information on diseases, conditions, medications, symptoms, healthy living, and more.

familydoctor.org

American Academy of Pediatrics (AAP)
Go straight to the Parenting Corner for advice on choosing a physician, immunizations, child development, safety and injury prevention, and more.

www.aap.org

Centers for Disease Control and Prevention
This is the place for official government health data and recommendations for kids from birth to age 20. You will find interactive tools, charts, growth tables, recommended vaccinations, and information on infectious and chronic diseases, injuries, disabilities, and environmental health threats.

www.cdc.gov

KidsHealth
Here you'll find practical, easy-to-read articles on a range of diseases and chronic conditions. There are also doctor-approved resources and information. The site is divided into unique areas for parents, children, and teens.

www.kidshealth.org

U.S. Department of Health and Human Services Office of Disease Prevention and Health Promotion
Check out this site with your kids! Includes games, contests, pointers on how to surf the Net safely and create personal sites, plus information on substance abuse, safety, and more.
　　www.healthfinder.gov/kids/

▶ **For resources on nutrition and eating habits, check out:**

American Dietetic Association (ADA)
Get clear answers to your family's food and nutrition questions. The ADA does a great job of translating the science of nutrition into practical solutions for healthy living through fact sheets, reading lists, and interactive activities.
　　www.eatright.org

Harvard School of Public Health Nutrition Source
You'll find Harvard's respected Healthy Eating Pyramid here. This site also covers current news about diet and nutrition and provides tools to help you make smart choices about your diet and long-term health.
　　www.hsph.harvard.edu/nutritionsource/

U.S. Food and Drug Administration's Center for Food Safety and Applied Nutrition
There is excellent advice here on keeping food and supplements safe, nutritious, and wholesome. Check out the Kids, Teens, and Educators sections for interactive quizzes, coloring worksheets, and more.
　　www.cfsan.fda.gov

U.S. Department of Agriculture (USDA)
Climb the newly revamped food pyramid and explore the latest dietary guidelines for you and your kids. Enter age, gender, and physical activity level and get personalized recommendations on daily caloric intakes and nutritional needs.
mypyramid.gov

▶ **For resources on kids' fitness needs, check out:**

The Educated Sports Parent
Covers important youth sports issues from the parents' point of view, including gauging readiness for participation, specialization, overuse injuries, and being a parent-coach.
www.educatedsportsparent.com

Get Active Stay Active
Learn effective strategies to encourage middle- and high-schoolers to become more physically active. The site features tools that allow students to record and total up their physical activity minutes.
www.getactivestayactive.com

National Center on Physical Activity and Disability (NCPAD)
Packed with information on adapting games and sports for specific disabilities, and finding disability-conscious fitness facilities and recreation programs where you live.
www.ncpad.org

National Center for Sports Safety
Get tips on helping your young athlete play it safe on the court, rink, field, track, or in the water. Plus, find out how to be a Parent Ambassador for Sports Safety (PASS).
www.sportssafety.org

VerbNow
On this interactive website, tweens can chat with other tweens about everything from roller hockey and mountain-bike riding to sailing and croquet. The site is produced by the Centers for Disease Control and Prevention.
www.verbnow.com

▶ **For info on kids' social and emotional health, check out:**

AboutOurKids.org
Visit this site produced by the New York University Child Study Center and find articles relating to children's emotional and mental health.
www.aboutourkids.org

American Academy of Child & Adolescent Psychiatry
Learn more about identifying and treating developmental, behavioral, emotional, and mental disorders in children and adolescents.
www.aacap.org

National Mental Health Association
Access resources designed to help families increase their understanding of children's mental health disorders such as depression, bipolar disorders, anxiety disorders, and ADHD.
www.nmha.org

▶ **For tips on keeping kids safe, check out:**

American Red Cross
Provides all kinds of information on health and safety training, as well as volunteer opportunities in your area for your family.
www.redcross.org

National Highway Traffic Safety Administration
Use this site's national search engine to track down local groups in your area that offer safety inspections of infant/child car seat installation.
www.seatcheck.org

PBS Parents: Children and Media
Discover how TV, movies, advertising, computers, and video games can shape your child's development and what you can do to create a media-literate household.
www.pbs.org/parents/childrenandmedia/

Safe Kids Worldwide
You'll find tons of useful information here on how to keep your children safe, including tips, checklists, and fact sheets.
www.safekids.org

U.S. Consumer Product Safety Commission:
The Further Adventures of Kidd Safety
Have fun exploring this site with your kids. It includes information on bike and scooter safety, and playground safety, and offers a Brain Buster quiz to reinforce information.
www.cpsc.gov/kids/kidsafety/

U.S. Consumer Product Safety Commission:
Recalls and Product Safety News
Keeps you up to date on safety alerts and recalls for over 4,000 consumer products, and many are kid- and family-oriented.
www.cpsc.gov/cpscpub/prerel/prerel.html

► **And if you're looking for some fun sites to visit with your kids, check out:**

American Library Association Great Website for Kids
Explore this directory of kid-friendly websites selected by members of the American Library Association to assure high quality content.
www.ala.org/greatsites

Awesome Library
Browse or search thousands of sites in this directory, which includes sections for kids, teens, parents, librarians, teachers, and students.
www.awesomelibrary.org

BAM! Body and Mind
Join in the fun at this interactive kids' site from the Centers for Disease Control and Prevention. It uses games, quizzes, and other interactive features to teach children about making healthy choices.
www.bam.gov

Dibdabdoo
Search or browse for interesting, original content about all aspects of family life in this ad-free, noncommercial directory of websites designed for child-safe use.
www.dibdabdoo.com

Girlshealth.gov
Designed for girls aged 10 to 16, this site from the U.S. Department of Health and Human Services offers, reliable, useful information on the health issues they will face as they become young women, including tips on handling relationships with family and friends.
www.girlshealth.gov

How Stuff Works: The Body Channel
Help kids understand how their body works when it's healthy and what happens when it breaks down with dozens of illustrated articles.

health.howstuffworks.com/the-body-channel.htm

KidsClick!
Point your kids to fun, age-appropriate websites with this librarian-run site covering more than 600 subjects.

www.kidsclick.org

Yuckiest Site on the Internet
Explore a range of fascinatingly yucky science topics with your kids. The site includes a section on understanding the gross and cool human body.

www.yucky.com

Selected References

Associations of parental, birth, and early life characteristics with systolic blood pressure at 5 years of age: findings from the Mater University study of pregnancy and its outcomes. Lawlor, D. A., Najman, J. M., Sterne, J., Williams, G. M., Ebrahim, S., Davey Smith, G., *Circulation* 2004 Oct 19;110(16):2417–2423.

Cetaphil cleanser (nuvo lotion) cures head lice. Pearlman, D. L., *Pediatrics* 2005;116:1612.

Childhood cardiovascular risk factors and carotid vascular changes in adulthood: the Bogalusa Heart Study. Li, S., Chen, W., Srinivasan, S. R., Bond, M. G., Tang, R., Urbina, E. M., Berenson, G. S. *Journal of the American Medical Association* 2003 Nov 5;290(17):2271–2276.

A clinical perspective of attention-deficit/hyperactivity disorder into adulthood. Wilens, T. E., Dodson, W., *Journal of Clinical Psychiatry* 2004 Oct;65(10):1301–1313.

Current concepts: streptococcal infections of skin and soft tissues. Bisno, A. L., Stevens, D. L., *New England Journal of Medicine* 1996; 334:240–245.

Depressive symptoms in adolescence as predictors of early adulthood depressive disorders and maladjustment. Aalto-Setala, T., Marttunen, M., Tuulio-Henriksson, A., Poiko-lainen, K., Lonnqvist, J., *American Journal of Psychiatry* 2002 Jul;159(7):1235–1237.

Do parents understand immunizations? A national telephone survey. Gellin, B. G., Maibach, E. W., Marcuse, E. K. *Pediatrics* 2000 Nov;106(5):1097–1102.

Does low self-esteem predict health compromising behaviours among adolescents? Mcgee, R., Williams, S., *Journal of Adolescence* 2000 Oct;23(5):569–582.

Does pacifier use cause ear infections in young children? Hanafin, S., Griffiths, P., *British Journal of Community Nursing* 2002 Apr;7(4):206, 208–211.

Early reading acquisition and its relation to reading experience and ability ten years later. Cunningham, A. E., Stanovich, K. E., *Developmental Psychology* 1997 Nov;33(6):934–945.

Effects of seating position and appropriate restraint use on the risk of injury to children in motor vehicle crashes. Durbin, D. R., Chen, I., Smith, R., Elliott, M. R., Winston, F. K., *Pediatrics* 2005 Mar;115(3):e305–309.

Evaluating a model of parental influence on youth physical activity. Trost, S. G., Sallis, J. F., Pate, R. R., Freedson, P. S., Taylor, W. C., Dowda, M., *American Journal of Preventive Medicine* 2003 Nov;25(4):277–282.

Family-based behavioural intervention for obese children. Epstein, L. H., *International Journal of Obesity* 1996 Feb;20 Suppl 1:S14–21.

Five-year obesity incidence in the transition period between adolescence and adulthood: the National Longitudinal Study of Adolescent Health. Gordon-Larsen, P., Adair, L. S., Nelson, M. C., Popkin, B. M., *American Journal of Clinical Nutrition* 2004 Sep;80(3):569–575.

Fluorides in caries prevention and control: empiricism or science. Ten, C. JM, *Caries Research* 2004 May-Jun;38(3):254–257.

Heat stress from enclosed vehicles: moderate ambient temperatures cause significant temperature rise in enclosed vehicles. McLaren, C., Null, J., Quinn, J., *Pediatrics* 2005 Jul;116(1):109–112.

History of acute knee injury and osteoarthritis of the knee: a prospective epidemiological assessment. The Clearwater Osteoarthritis Study. Wilder, F. V., Hall, B. J., Barrett, J. P. Jr., Lemrow, N. B., *Osteoarthritis and Cartilage* 2002 Aug;10(8):611–616.

Home syrup of ipecac use does not reduce emergency department use or improve outcome. Bond, G. R., *Pediatrics* 2003 Nov;112(5):1061–1064.

Identification and remediation of pediatric fluency and voice disorders. Baker, B. M., Blackwell, P. B., *Journal of Pediatric Health Care* 2004 Mar-Apr;18(2):87–94.

Inflammation, cardiovascular disease and destructive periodontal diseases. The evolving role of the dental profession. Craig R. G., *New York State Dental Journal* 2004 May-Jun; 70(5):22–26.

Life events, entrapments and arrested anger in depression. Gilbert, P., Gilbert, J., Irons, C., *Journal of Affective Disorders* 2004 Apr;79(1–3):149–160.

Lipid profile with paternal history of coronary heart disease before age 40. Bistritzer, T., Rosenzweig, L., Barr, J., Mayer, S., Lahat, E., Faibel, H., Schlesinger, Z., Aladjem, M., *Archives of Disease in Childhood* 1995 Jul;73(1):62–65.

Longitudinal physical activity and sedentary behavior trends: adolescence to adulthood. Gordon-Larsen, P., Nelson, M. C., Popkin, B. M., *American Journal of Preventive Medicine* 2004 Nov;27(4):277–283.

Longitudinal trends in race/ethnic disparities in leading health indicators from adolescence to young adulthood. Harris, K. M., Gordon-Larsen, P., Chantala, K., Udry, J. R., *Archives of Pediatric and Adolescent Medicine* 2006 Jan;160(1):74–81.

Matched analysis of parents' and children's attitudes and practices towards motor vehicle and bicycle safety: an important information gap. Ehrlich, P. F., Helmkamp, J. C., Williams, J. M., Haque, A., Furbee, P. M., *Injury Control and Safety Promotion* 2004 Mar;11(1):23–28.

Metabolic syndrome variables at low levels in childhood are beneficially associated with adulthood cardiovascular risk: the Bogalusa Heart Study. Chen, W., Srinivasan, S. R., Li, S., Xu, J., Berenson, G. S., *Diabetes Care* 2005 Jan;28(1):126–131.

The observed effects of teenage passengers on the risky driving behavior of teenage drivers. Simons-Morton, B., Lerner, N., Singer, J., *Accident Analysis and Prevention* 2005 Nov;37(6):973–982.

Pacifier as a risk factor for acute otitis media: a randomized, controlled trial of parental counseling. Nimela, M., Pihakari, O., Pokka, T., Uhari, M., *Pediatrics* 2000 Sep;106(3):483–488.

Pacifier use in children: a review of recent literature. Adair, S. M., *Pediatric Dentistry* 2003 Sep-Oct;25(5):449–458.

Parental eating attitudes and the development of obesity in children. The Framingham Children's Study. Hood, M. Y., Moore, L. L., Sundarajan-Ramamurti, A., Singer, M., Cupples, L. A., Ellison, R. C., *International Journal of Obesity and Related Metabolic Disorders* 2000 Oct;24(10):1319–1325.

Parenting style and adolescent's reaction to conflict: is there a relationship? Miller, J. M., DiIorio, C., Dudley, W., *Journal of Adolescence Health* 2002 Dec;31(6):463–468.

Pediatric restraint use in motor vehicle collisions: reduction of deaths without contribution to injury. Tyroch, A. H., Kaups, K. L., Sue, L. P., O'Donnell-Nicol, S., *Archives of Surgery* 2000 Oct;135(10):1173–1176.

Physical activity and biological risk factors clustering in pediatric population. Ribeiro, J. C., Guerra, S., Oliveira, J., Teixeira-Pinto, A., Twisk, J. W., Duarte, J. A., Mota J., *Preventive Medicine* 2004 Sep;39(3):596–601.

Physical activity as a preventive measure for coronary heart disease risk factors in early childhood. Saakslahti, A., Numminen, P., Varstala, V., Helenius, H., Tammi, A., Viikari, J., Valimaki, I., *Scandinavian Journal of Medicine & Science in Sports* 2004 Jun;14(3):143–149.

Prospective risk factors for alcohol misuse in late adolescence. Ellickson, S. L., Tucker, J. S., Klein, D. J., McGuigan, K. A., *Journal of Studies on Alcohol* 2001 Nov;62(6):773–782.

The relation of obesity throughout life to carotid intima-media thickness in adulthood: the Bogalusa Heart Study. Freedman, D. S., Dietz, W. H., Tang, R., Mensah, G. A.,

Bond, M. G., Urbina, E. M., Srinivasan, S., Berenson, G. S., *International Journal of Obesity and Related Metababolic Disorders* 2004 Jan;28(1):159–166.

The relationship between physical activity and self-image and problem behaviour among adolescents. Kirkcaldy, B. D., Shephard, R. J., Siefen, R. G., *Social Psychiatry and Psychiatric Epidemiology* 2002 Nov;37(11):544–550.

Relationship of physical activity and television watching with body weight and level of fatness among children: results from the Third National Health and Nutrition Examination Survey. Andersen, R. E., Crespo, C. J., Bartlett, S. J., Cheskin, L. J., Pratt, M., *Journal of the American Medical Association* 1998 Mar 25;279(12):938–942.

Sleep problems in early childhood and early onset of alcohol and other drug use in adolescence. Wong, M. M., Brower, K. J., Fitzgerald, H. E., Zucker, R. A., *Alcoholism, Clinical and Experimental Research* 2004 Apr;28(4):578–587.

Stress burden and the lifetime incidence of psychiatric disorder in young adults: racial and ethnic contrasts. Turner, R. J., Lloyd, D. A., *Archives of General Psychiatry* 2004 May;61(5):481–488.

Summertime sun protection used by adults for their children. Robinson, J. K., Rigel, D. S., Amonette, R. A., *Journal of the American Academy of Dermatology* 2000 May;42(5 Pt 1):746–753.

Television watching, energy intake, and obesity in U.S. children: results from the third National Health and Nutrition Examination Survey, 1988–1994. Crespo, C. J., Smit, E., Troiano, R. P., Bartlett, S. J., Macera, C. A., Andersen, R. E., *Archives of Pediatrics & Adolescent Medicine* 2001 Mar;155(3):360–365.

Use of a dummy (pacifier) during sleep and risk of sudden infant death syndrome (SIDS): population based case-control study. Li, D. K., Willinger, M., Pettiti, D. B., Oduli, R., Liu, L., Hoffman, H. J., *BMJ* 2006 Jan 7;332(7532):18–22.

Weighing the risks of treatment versus nontreatment in pediatric asthma. Spahn, J. D., Covar, R. A., *Pediatric Clinics of North America* 2003 Jun;50(3):677–695.

Weight management through lifestyle modification for the prevention and management of type 2 diabetes: rationale and strategies. Klein, S., Sheard, N. F., Pi-Sunyer, X., Daly, A., Wylie-Rosett, J., Kulkarni, K., Clark, N. G., American Diabetes Association, North American Association for the Study of Obesity, American Society for Clinical Nutrition, *American Journal of Clinical Nutrition* 2004 Aug;80(2):257–263.

What predicts good relationships with parents in adolescence and partners in adult life: findings from the 1958 British birth cohort. Flouri, E., Buchanan, A., *Journal of Family Psychology* 2002 Jun;16(2):186–198.

ACKNOWLEDGMENTS

As everyone who sets out to create a book quickly discovers, it takes a huge number of people to actually do it. I'm grateful to:

- The editorial talent at RealAge, who pored over every page, especially Val Weaver and Carol Valdez. I hope they had as much fun working with me as I did with them. I can't forget Charlie Silver, the vision behind RealAge, Jennifer Perciballi, and agent Candice Fuhrman—without them, I might never have had this opportunity.
- The publishing pros at HarperCollins, particularly my editor, Kathryn Huck, and Joe Tessitore, for believing in me and in this book.
- My partners at Carnegie Hill Pediatrics: Stephanie Freilich, MD, Harold Raucher, MD, Neal Kotin, MD, and Barry Stein, MD. They not only encouraged me, they allowed me the time to pursue a book that would help parents and kids take charge of their health—a book that would help improve the future lives of far more children than I could ever possibly see in my office.
- My parents, Leila and Sheldon Brooks, for always encouraging me to go after my dreams—professional and per-

sonal—and for teaching me the importance of family and unconditional love. I would not be able to wear so many hats without a mom who's always been there to pinch-hit for me, and who's always seen babysitting as a pleasure, never a chore.

- My sitters, Barbara Sutherland and Keith Hand, who over the years have spent so much time with my family that they are family. When I have to be away from my children, in order to work helping other kids/families, they give me peace of mind.

- My sisters and best friends, Allison and Suzanne, whom I can count on to be there for me in the best and worst of times.

- And of course, my husband, David, who is not only a wonderful partner—endlessly supportive, encouraging, and patient, especially during this past year when my normally hectic schedule hit overdrive, thanks to the book—but who is also an unbelievable hands-on dad. When the kids are with him, time never stands still. They're skiing or hiking or building a bonfire or heading out to pick apples or tumbling through a pick-up football game. (And our children don't have a clue how fit they're getting from all this homemade fun!)

- Last and best are my three wonderful, uniquely different children, Noah, Eric, and Emily—I never fail to get a smile on my face from just thinking about them and knowing that I will always be their mom.

INDEX

R   r